GW00702120

Individualized Approaches to
Diabetes
Nutrition Therapy
CASE STUDIES

Individualized Approaches to
Diabetes
Nutrition Therapy
CASE STUDIES

Carolyn Leontos, MS, RD, CDE
Patti Geil, MS, RD, FADA, CDE

American Diabetes Association
Cure • Care • Commitment

Director, Book Publishing, John Fedor; *Associate Director, Professional Books,* Christine B. Welch; *Editor,* Joyce Raynor; *Production Manager,* Peggy M. Rote; *Composition,* Circle Graphics, Inc.; *Cover Design,* Koncept, Inc.; *Printer,* Hamilton Printing Company

©2002 by the American Diabetes Association, Inc. All Rights Reserved. No part of this publication may be reproduced or transmitted in any form or by any means, electronic or mechanical, including duplication, recording, or any information storage and retrieval system, without the prior written permission of the American Diabetes Association.

Printed in the United States of America
1 3 5 7 9 10 8 6 4 2

The suggestions and information contained in this publication are generally consistent with the *Clinical Practice Recommendations* and other policies of the American Diabetes Association, but they do not represent the policy or position of the Association or any of its boards or committees. Reasonable steps have been taken to ensure the accuracy of the information presented. However, the American Diabetes Association cannot ensure the safety or efficacy of any product or service described in this publication. Individuals are advised to consult a physician or other appropriate health care professional before undertaking any diet or exercise program or taking any medication referred to in this publication. Professionals must use and apply their own professional judgment, experience, and training and should not rely solely on the information contained in this publication before prescribing any diet, exercise, or medication. The American Diabetes Association—its officers, directors, employees, volunteers, and members—assumes no responsibility or liability for personal or other injury, loss, or damage that may result from the suggestions or information in this publication.

⊗ The paper in this publication meets the requirements of the ANSI Standard Z39.48-1992 (permanence of paper).

ADA titles may be purchased for business or promotional use or for special sales. To purchase this book in large quantities, or for custom editions of this book with your logo, contact Lee Romano Sequeira, Special Sales & Promotions, at the address below, or at Lromano@diabetes.org or call 703-299-2046.

American Diabetes Association
1701 North Beauregard Street
Alexandria, Virginia 22311

Library of Congress Cataloging-in-Publication Data

Leontos, Carolyn.
   Individualized approaches to diabetes nutrition therapy : case studies / Carolyn Leontos and Patti Geil.
      p. cm.
   Includes bibliographical references.
   ISBN 1-58040-167-8 (pbk. : alk. paper)
     1. Diabetes—Diet therapy—Case studies. I. Geil, Patti Bazel. II. Title.

RC662 .L465 2002
616.4′620654—dc21

                            2002026102

Contents

Dedication

We dedicate this book to our patients, who over the years have taught us more than we are capable of teaching them, and to our professional colleagues, who labored to develop the Nutrition Practice Guidelines that make it possible for us to consistently provide our patients with quality care.

Introduction

Nutrition recommendations for individuals with diabetes have evolved over the years from starvation diets and "no concentrated sweets" to controlled carbohydrate counting. And because people differ, finding the optimal approach for each individual is the challenge for the registered dietitian (RD). We can find answers by using Nutrition Practice Guidelines (NPGs) to determine what is best for each person.

What are NPGs? They are systematically developed statements designed to assist practitioner decisions about appropriate health care for specific clinical circumstances (1). They outline the process the professional should consider in providing medical nutrition therapy to individuals with type 1 diabetes, type 2 diabetes, and gestational diabetes mellitus. They are not a "cookbook approach" but do offer a step-by-step process. Following a predetermined process helps the RD remember to include each step and not omit anything important.

Practice guidelines work. When the NPGs were field tested, results showed that blood glucose control improved and patients reduced their A1C by 1% on average (1).

The process includes the following five steps: 1) assessment, 2) goal setting and nutrition care plan, 3) intervention, 4) documentation and communication, and 5) evaluation and re-assessment. Others have adapted the NPGs to their practice setting. They use: 1) assessment, 2) intervention, 3) goal setting, and 4) communication (2).

An RD who uses the NPGs follows a systematic process. The first step is assessment. Assessments are based on referral data, which includes medical history, medications, and laboratory data as well as information provided by the patient and family members. Figure 1 is a patient questionnaire for type 1 or type 2 diabetes adapted from Appendix 16 of the *Nutrition Practice Guidelines for Type 1 and Type 2 Diabetes* (1) that is an excellent tool to help gather this data. Other team members often provide valuable information as well. A complete nutrition assessment includes all past nutrition education, or lack thereof, as well as the patient's perception of that experience. It establishes rapport, which is particularly helpful in the goal setting stage. The professional needs to determine the way in which the patient learns. It is important to consider health beliefs, attitudes, behaviors, and specific food habits that may be unique to your patient. Whether family members are supportive may not be obvious. Literacy level, visual status, disabilities, and socio-economic status are all important factors in the assessment.

A comprehensive assessment is a crucial step in providing individualized diabetes nutrition therapy. The assessment allows the professional to tailor the intervention and the diabetes nutrition therapy to the individual. The RD cannot begin to establish goals or determine a care plan and intervention without a sound basis. The assessment provides the basis of nutrition therapy and self-management training. Figure 2 shows a nutrition assessment form adapted from Appendix 6 of the *Nutrition Practice Guidelines for Type 1 and Type 2 Diabetes* (1).

The second step is to establish goals and determine the nutrition care plan. When attempting to establish goals, the RD must distinguish between short- and long-term goals and between the goals of the patient and those of the health care

FIGURE 1: Diabetes Patient Questionnaire

1. When were you first told you had diabetes? _____

   Have you had previous instruction on diet? ☐ yes ☐ no

   If yes, who provided the instruction? _____

   When was this done? _____

   Do you have a meal plan? ☐ yes ☐ no

   If yes, how many calories? _____

   How much of the time are you able to follow it?

           0%–25%   25%–50%   50%–75%   75%–100%

2. Have you been told to follow any other diet restrictions? ☐ yes ☐ no

   If yes, please check which restrictions.

   ☐ low calorie ☐ low cholesterol ☐ low salt/sodium ☐ low protein

   ☐ low fat ☐ high fiber ☐ other: _____

3. Has your weight changed in the last year? ☐ yes ☐ no

   If yes, describe the change. _____

   What is your height? _____

   What is your usual weight? _____

   What would you like to weigh? _____

   What has been your highest weight? _____

   If you now weigh less than your highest weight, how did you lose the weight?

   _____

4. Rate your appetite: ☐ good ☐ fair ☐ poor

   Do you have any eating or digestion problems?

   ☐ chewing ☐ swallowing ☐ stomachache ☐ diarrhea

   ☐ constipation ☐ other: _____

5. What are your usual work hours? _____

6. What is your usual eating schedule and what did you eat in the last 24 hours?

   Time _____ Breakfast or first meal _____

   _____

   Time _____ Snack _____

   Time _____ Lunch or second meal _____

   _____

   Time _____ Snack _____

   Time _____ Dinner or third meal _____

   _____

   Time _____ Snack _____

7. Who prepares the meals? ☐ self ☐ spouse ☐ roommate ☐ other

   Are there any special considerations in family meal planning? _____

   _____

(continued)

FIGURE 1: Diabetes Patient Questionnaire (*continued*)

8. How often each week do you eat in restaurants, cafeterias, or away from home?

   Breakfast _____ x/week   Lunch _____ x/week   Dinner _____ x/week

   What type of restaurant? _____

9. Do you drink alcohol?   ☐ beer   ☐ wine   ☐ liquor

   How often? _____   How much? _____

10. How many times a week do you eat these foods?

    regular soda pop   _____ x/week

    sweet roll/pastries   _____ x/week

    candy, candy bars   _____ x/week

    desserts—pie, cake   _____ x/week

    ice cream/other   _____ x/week

    frozen desserts   _____ x/week

    cookies   _____ x/week

    other _____   _____ x/week

11. Do you take vitamins or any other nutrition supplement?   ☐ yes   ☐ no

    If yes, please list. _____

12. Do you exercise now?   ☐ yes   ☐ no

    If yes, what do you do? _____

    How frequently?   _____ x/week

    If no, what exercise would you consider?   ☐ walking   ☐ exercise class

    ☐ other: _____

    Do you have any limitations on exercise?   ☐ yes   ☐ no

    If yes, please describe. _____

13. If the doctor recommends a change in your current eating habits, would this be difficult?   ☐ yes   ☐ no

    If yes, why? _____

14. What eating concerns do you have? _____

    _____

15. What would you like to know more about?

    ☐ weight loss   ☐ exercise

    ☐ eating out   ☐ label reading

    ☐ alcohol use   ☐ sweeteners

    ☐ other: _____

16. What do you hope to accomplish or gain from this appointment?

    I would like to:

    ☐ improve blood glucose   ☐ get more information

    ☐ improve eating habits   ☐ start exercising

    ☐ lose weight   ☐ lower cholesterol/triglycerides

    ☐ other: _____

Adapted with permission from *ADA MNT Evidence Based Guides for Practice: Nutrition Practice Guidelines for Type 1 and Type 2 Diabetes Mellitus*, Chicago, IL: The American Dietetic Association, 2001.

provider. Goals for both parties should be reasonable, attainable, and measurable. Examples of measurable behavioral goals can be found in each case study presented in this book. If the professional has established a good rapport with the patient, it is easier to negotiate attainable goals. Keep in mind that goals evolve and, with time, need to be evaluated and frequently renegotiated as circumstances change.

Once goals are established, the nutrition care plan can be established. An analysis of the assessment data helps you determine attitudes and beliefs about diabetes. It also gives the RD insight into the patient's ability and motivation to make the lifestyle changes necessary to manage their disease. Prochaska et al.'s (3) Transtheoretical Model for behavioral change outlines the stages of change—precontemplation, contemplation, preparation, action, and maintenance—and allows the RD to understand and help the patient at each of the stages.

Understanding these stages, and the fact that people move through them in an unsystematic fashion, helps to minimize unrealistic expectations. If the patient believes the health care professional is in charge of health care decisions and has never been introduced to the concept of self-management, it is naïve to think she or he will be willing to take charge of their own health. However, it is appropriate at this stage to introduce the concept of self-management as food for thought.

The third step is to implement the intervention. According to Holler and Pastors (4), intervention refers to the diabetes educator's activities, specifically those that facilitate or support the patient's diabetes nutrition self-management plan. Education, providing accurate and timely information to the patient, is key at this step. However, the role of the educator goes beyond merely supplying facts. The educator is a counselor and a coach, helping the patient understand the disease and cope with its implications. The educator is a partner with the patient in disease management, helping him or her discover how they may be motivated to change behavior.

Once the nutrition prescription has been established, meal planning survival skills can be taught. Select the appropriate

FIGURE 2: Diabetes Nutrition Assessment Form

Name _____ Age _____ Date _____

Diagnosis of diabetes _____ Present diabetes treatment _____ Dietitian _____

Medical history _____ Other medications _____ Chart # _____

Physician _____

Lab Data   **Target Goals**

A1C _____ BG _____   Target BGs _____ mg/dl to _____ mg/dl

Cholesterol _____ HDL-C _____   Target A1C _____ %

Triglycerides _____ LDL-C _____

BP _____ Microalbumin _____   Other _____

SMBG: Frequency _____ Times of day _____   Method _____

Medical clearance for exercise: Y / N _____ **Exercise limitations** _____

Time	Bkfst	Snack	Lunch	Snack	Dinner	Snack	Total servings/ day	CHO (g)	Protein (g)	Fat (g)	Calories
Starch								15	3	1	80
Fruit								15			60
Milk								12	8	1	90
Veg								5	2		25
Meat/Sub									7	5(3)	75(55)
Fat										5	45
Other							Total g				Total =
							Calories %Kcal	×4	×4	×9	

Ht _____ (_____ %) Wt history _____
Wt _____ (_____ %) Reasonable wt _____
Estimated calorie expenditure + Activity factor = Total calorie needs _____

History

Occupation _____ Hours worked _____
Lives with _____ Meal preparation _____
Hypoglycemia _____ Eating out _____
Schedule changes/weekends/school schedule _____
Exercise: type/frequency _____
Appetite/GI problems/allergies/intolerances _____
Vitamin and mineral supplements _____
Psychosocial/economic _____

Assessment

_____
_____
_____
_____

Goals (nutrition/exercise/SMBG)

_____
_____

© 1996 International Diabetes Center, Minneapolis, USA. Used with permission.

meal-planning approach (see Resources, p. 71) with the understanding that this may change as the patient's understanding of the disease and motivation to self-manage evolve.

The fourth step is to document in the medical record and communicate to other members of the health care team. Clearly document both clinical and behavioral goals, including nutrition prescription, meal planning approach, and educational topics covered, after the first visit. The medical nutrition therapy protocol components of the NPGs (1) have nutrition progress notes that can be used for documentation; Figure 3 shows an adaptation of this form that is referred to in the following case studies and that you may find useful. After subsequent visits, you will want to document and communicate patient acceptance and understanding, behavioral changes made, and plans for ongoing care to the patient's primary care giver (usually the referral source) and other team members (1). Written documentation can be shared with the patient to demonstrate their progress to them and encourage further efforts.

Finally, the fifth step is to evaluate and reassess. Measurable goals help to make evaluation a straightforward task. If initial goals have not been met, they may need to be changed or renegotiated. Presenting this process as merely a course correction makes it less threatening to the patient. If initial goals have been met, new reasonable, attainable, and measurable goals may be set.

Through case studies, this book demonstrates the use of NPGs to simplify nutrition practice, help ensure success for patients, and produce outcomes that can be easily documented. In Case 4, we provide examples of how we complete the forms we use for assessment and documentation, in this instance for a type 2 diabetes patient being treated with an oral hypoglycemic agent. The Resources (pages 71–74) provide references for the professional and useful publications for patients.

1. American Dietetic Association: *ADA MNT Evidence Based Guides for Practice: Nutrition Practice Guidelines for Type 1 and Type 2 Diabetes Mellitus.* Chicago, IL: American Dietetic Association, 2001.

2. Franz MJ, Reader D, Monk A: *Implementing Group and Individual Medical Nutrition Therapy for Diabetes.* Alexandria, VA: American Diabetes Association, 2002.
3. Prochaska J, Redding C, Evers K: *The Transtheoretical Model and Stages of Change.* 2nd ed. R. Health Behavior and Health Education Theory, and Practice, ed. 1997, San Francisco: Jossey-Bass, Inc., 1997, p. 60–84.
4. Holler H, Pastors JG: *Diabetes Medical Nutrition Therapy.* Chicago, IL: American Dietetic Association, and Alexandria, VA: American Diabetes Association, 1997.

FIGURE 3: Diabetes Nutrition Progress Notes

Client's Name: _____ Phone Number: _____ Medical Record #: _____

DOB: _____ Gender: _____

Other Diagnosis: _____ Ethnic Background (Optional): _____ Referring Physician: _____

Encounters outcome	Intervention provided to meet goal (intervention = self-management training plus client verbalizes/demonstrates)				Outcomes of Medical Nutrition Therapy (MNT) Goal reached (√ indicates goal reached, follow with number 1–5 as indicated* e.g. √–3, √–5)			
Encounters	1 (60–90 min)	2 (30–45 min)	3 (30–45 min)	4 (30–45 min)	Date: ___ 1	Date: ___ 2	Date: ___ 3	Date: ___ 4
Clinical Outcomes					Value	Value	Value	Value
Preprandial blood glucose (md/dL)								
Bedtime blood glucose (mg/dL)								
A1C (%)								
SMBG, % in target range								
LDL-C (mg/dL)								
HDL-C (mg/dL)								
Triglycerides (mg/dL)								
Microalbumin (mcg/24 hr)								
Blood pressure					___/___	___/___	___/___	___/___
Height ___ Weight/BMI								
Hypo/hyperglycemic episodes					x/mo	x/mo	x/mo	x/mo
MNT Goal: ___ kcal ___ g CHO total ___ g CHO/meal ___ % Fat					___ kcal ___ g CHO total ___ g CHO meals ___ % fat	___ kcal ___ g CHO total ___ g CHO meals ___ % fat	___ kcal ___ g CHO total ___ g CHO meals ___ % fat	___ kcal ___ g CHO total ___ g CHO meals ___ % fat
Adhere to appropriate meal pattern, exercise, and medication treatment; plan to maintain blood glucose and lipids within normal limits								

Behavioral Outcomes

• Eats meals/snacks at appropriate times		1 2 3 4 5	1 2 3 4 5	1 2 3 4 5	1 2 3 4 5
• Chooses food and amounts per meal plan		1 2 3 4 5	1 2 3 4 5	1 2 3 4 5	1 2 3 4 5
• Verbalizes sick-day management skills		1 2 3 4 5	1 2 3 4 5	1 2 3 4 5	1 2 3 4 5
• Manages signs and symptoms of hypoglycemia		1 2 3 4 5	1 2 3 4 5	1 2 3 4 5	1 2 3 4 5
• Accurately reads food labels		1 2 3 4 5	1 2 3 4 5	1 2 3 4 5	1 2 3 4 5
• Uses modified or modifies recipes to reduce total fat/saturated fat/sodium		1 2 3 4 5	1 2 3 4 5	1 2 3 4 5	1 2 3 4 5
• Uses healthy cooking techniques		1 2 3 4 5	1 2 3 4 5	1 2 3 4 5	1 2 3 4 5
• Selects appropriately from restaurant menu		1 2 3 4 5	1 2 3 4 5	1 2 3 4 5	1 2 3 4 5
• Participates in aerobic activity per exercise prescription		1 2 3 4 5 __x/wk __min	1 2 3 4 5 __x/wk __min	1 2 3 4 5 __x/wk __min	1 2 3 4 5 __x/wk __min
• Limits alcohol use to 1–2 drinks/day		1 2 3 4 5 __svg	1 2 3 4 5 __svg	1 2 3 4 5 __svg	1 2 3 4 5 __svg
• Verbalizes importance of smoking cessation		1 2 3 4 5	1 2 3 4 5	1 2 3 4 5	1 2 3 4 5
• Modifies medication/food for activity/lifestyle		1 2 3 4 5	1 2 3 4 5	1 2 3 4 5	1 2 3 4 5
• Verbalizes potential food/drug interaction Drug		1 2 3 4 5 __ dose __ dose	1 2 3 4 5 __ dose __ dose	1 2 3 4 5 __ dose __ dose	1 2 3 4 5 __ dose __ dose
*Overall Compliance Potential**					
Comprehension		1 2 3 4 5	1 2 3 4 5	1 2 3 4 5	1 2 3 4 5
Receptivity		1 2 3 4 5	1 2 3 4 5	1 2 3 4 5	1 2 3 4 5
Adherence		1 2 3 4 5	1 2 3 4 5	1 2 3 4 5	1 2 3 4 5

Intervention: D Discussed, R Reinforced/Reviewed, ≠ Not reviewed, Outcome achieved, N/A Not applicable.
* Key for Compliance Potential and Overall Adherence Potential: 1=Never demonstrated, 2=Rarely demonstrated, 3=Sometimes demonstrated, 4=Often demonstrated, 5=Consistently demonstrated.

INITIAL ENCOUNTER

Date: _____

Beginning Time: _____ Ending Time: _____ Total Minutes: _____

Comments: _____

_____

_____

_____

_____

Client Goals: _____

Material Provided: _____

Next Visit: _____ RD Signature: _____

FOLLOWUP ENCOUNTER

Date: _____

Beginning Time: _____ Ending Time: _____ Total Minutes: _____

Comments: _____

_____

_____

_____

_____

Client Goals: _____

Material Provided: _____

Next Visit: _____ RD Signature: _____

FOLLOWUP ENCOUNTER

Date: _____

Beginning Time: _____ Ending Time: _____ Total Minutes: _____

Comments: _____

_____

_____

_____

_____

Client Goals: _____

Material Provided: _____

Next Visit: _____ RD Signature: _____

FOLLOWUP ENCOUNTER

Date: _____

Beginning Time: _____ Ending Time: _____ Total Minutes: _____

Comments: _____

_____

_____

_____

_____

Client Goals: _____

Material Provided: _____

Next Visit: _____ RD Signature: _____

Adapted with permission from *ADA MNT Evidence Based Guides for Practice: Nutrition Practice Guidelines for Type 1 and Type 2 Diabetes Mellitus*, Chicago, IL: The American Dietetic Association, 2001.

CASE

1

Managing Prediabetes with Medical Nutrition Therapy and Physical Activity

SF is a 54-year-old African American female referred to the RD for medical nutrition therapy for prediabetes.

Assessment

SF asked for a referral to see the RD after a visit to her family practice physician confirmed her suspicions that she had prediabetes. The week before her visit, the RD obtained SF's medical record and reviewed it for pertinent clinical assessment information. The RD noted that SF made an appointment with her physician after she attended a health fair at her church and took the American Diabetes Association Risk Test for Diabetes. SF found that she had several of the risk factors for diabetes, including being overweight, having a sibling with diabetes, and being between 45 and 64 years of age. Because she is African American, SF also noted that diabetes was more common in individuals of her ethnic background. On further review of the medical record, the RD noted that SF had two fasting plasma glucose tests in the past two weeks; the first result was 124 mg/dl and the second was 118 mg/dl, confirming the diagnosis of prediabetes. SF had two additional medical problems—hypertension and high cholesterol—both of which were controlled by medication. Additionally, SF had had an exercise stress test.

At the initial clinic visit, which was scheduled for 90 minutes, SF weighed 166 lb and at 61 inches tall had a BMI of 31.4. She expressed a desire to lose "at least 40 lb" and indicated she was eager to prevent or delay the development of type 2 diabetes. The RD congratulated SF on her assertive approach to good health and completed a more thorough lifestyle assessment. SF is widowed, lives alone, and does not work outside her home. Her social life revolves around her church services and fellowship on Wednesday evenings and Sundays. SF stays busy babysitting and "running after" her grandchildren but has no regular program of physical activity.

Her diet recall reveals a typical day's intake of 2300 calories with approximately 345 grams of carbohydrate. SF has never been much of a breakfast eater, sometimes waiting until lunch to have her first meal of the day. However, she usually sipped on several glasses of sugared iced tea throughout the morning and had a few cookies as a snack if her grandchildren were with her and it was time for their midmorning snack. Lunch generally was around noon and often consisted of leftovers from supper the evening before: a meat such as pork chops, two vegetables such as fried okra or green bean/mushroom soup casserole, potatoes of some type, biscuits, and sweet potato pie for dessert. SF didn't usually snack in the afternoon, and her supper was similar to lunch, perhaps with larger portions. On most nights before bed, SF enjoyed having another serving of dessert. However, on Wednesday and Sunday evenings, SF attended a potluck supper after church services and regularly ate the high-calorie, high-fat foods that tempted her at those times. SF did not drink alcohol, but she did smoke ½ pack of cigarettes per day. She took no other medications, vitamins, or herbal supplements in addition to what had been prescribed for her hypertension and hypercholesterolemia.

Goal Setting and Nutrition Care Plan

The RD discussed the diagnosis of prediabetes with SF, noting that SF's blood glucose levels were higher than normal but not high enough for the diagnosis of diabetes. The RD stressed that intervening at this stage may actually allow SF's elevated blood glucose levels to return to the normal range, preventing or delaying the diagnosis of type 2 diabetes. Although SF wanted to lose a significant amount of weight, the RD counseled her that a modest weight loss of 5–10% of body weight (8–16 lb in her case) could make a clinically significant difference. The RD reinforced SF's physician's advice that lifestyle changes such as healthy food choices, along with moderate exercise such as walking 30 minutes per day, 5 days a week, are the best treatment for prediabetes. For this session, SF set a goal of measuring her actual food and beverage intake and writing it down for three days before her next clinic appointment; she was to include at least one weekend day on her recall sheet. SF also planned to investigate exercise programs that may be sponsored by her church and enroll in a smoking cessation program.

Intervention

To increase SF's awareness of proper portion sizes and the amount of carbohydrate she was consuming, the RD reviewed *The First Step in Diabetes Meal Planning* with SF. The RD marked each section of the food pyramid with the number of servings to total approximately 1800 calories per day: 7 servings of grains, beans and starchy vegetables; 4 servings of vegetables; 3 servings of fruits; 2–3 servings of milk and yogurt; 2 servings of meat and meat substitutes; and very limited amounts of fats, sweets, and alcohol. SF was surprised to note that her portion sizes of most foods had been quite a bit larger than those suggested. She agreed to substitute tea sweetened with a sugar substitute for the sugared iced tea she usually drank. The RD suggested that SF begin to try to consume a small first meal each morning and to spread her carbohydrate intake throughout the day by including small between-meal snacks of foods from the diabetes food pyramid. SF agreed to begin making changes, and a return appointment was set for three weeks later.

> **Initial visit: Goal setting**
> 1. I will measure my food and beverage intake for three days, record the amounts, and bring the records to my next clinic appointment.
> 2. I will investigate local exercise programs.
> 3. I will enroll in a smoking cessation program.
> 4. I will substitute sugar-free iced tea for sweetened tea.

Documentation and Communication

The RD completed a nutrition progress note with details such as relevant history, risk factors, assessment, intervention plan, and rational for treatment as well as actual time spent with the patient. She placed her note in SF's medical record and sent a copy to SF's physician, noting that a return appointment had been set.

Follow-Up Visit (3 weeks after first visit, 30 minutes)

At her three-week follow-up visit, SF had lost 2 lb. Although SF was discouraged with the small amount of weight she had lost, the RD told her how pleased she was with her progress. SF brought her diet recall sheet to her follow-up visit, again noting that portion sizes were a major issue. She had been able to make some healthy changes in her food choices, such as switching to sugar-free tea and spacing her calories and carbohydrate throughout the day. SF had not yet enrolled in a smoking cessation program, but she had joined a "mall walkers" program sponsored by her church, which enabled her to begin walking for physical activity three days per week.

3-week follow-up visit: Goal status
1. Achieved goal.
2. Has begun a mall walkers program three days per week.
3. Did not complete goal.
4. Achieved goal.

The bountiful potluck suppers at church were still a difficult challenge for SF, especially with the approaching holiday season. The RD suggested that SF bring a lower-fat version of one of her favorite dishes to holiday events so there would always be something she could choose on the table. The RD also advised SF to have a small snack before leaving for church, so she wouldn't be famished at the meal afterward and taught her to scan the buffet for healthy choices before she began eating. SF agreed to concentrate more on the people and fellowship at the events rather than the food. The RD suggested cookbooks for SF to use as a resource for modifying some of her favorite ethnic dishes, including *The New Soul Food Cookbook for People with Diabetes* (see Resources).

SF decided that before her next visit she would try to modify two or three recipes and walk at least four days a week.

New goals
1. I will modify three favorite recipes into lower-fat and lower-carbohydrate versions.
2. I will walk four days per week.
3. I will enroll in a smoking cessation program.

Documentation and Communication

The RD completed a nutrition progress note documenting the time she spent and delineating SF's progress to date including her weight loss. She placed her note in SF's medical record and sent a copy to the referring physician, noting an appointment had been set for six weeks later.

Evaluation and Reassessment

SF returned in six weeks for her third appointment with the RD. Her medical record showed that a fasting blood glucose test two weeks earlier had results of 108 mg/dl. Today's weight was 160 lb, showing a total weight loss of 6 lb since her initial appointment nine weeks ago. She was walking for 30 minutes four or five days a week. SF reported that she had modified her sweet potato pie recipe and taken this lower calorie version to a church potluck. After she received rave reviews on her pie, she told her friends that it had been modified. This success motivated her to try to reduce fat, sugar, and salt in other recipes. SF had made excellent progress. The RD encouraged her to continue her efforts and to call if she had any questions or problems. The RD cautioned SF not to set unrealistic goals and also said that if SF feels she needs additional help, especially after the holiday season, in meeting her nutrition and weight loss goals to call for an appointment.

Managing Type 2 Diabetes with Medical Nutrition Therapy and Physical Activity

MG is a 45-year-old Hispanic female referred to the RD for medical nutrition therapy for type 2 diabetes.

Assessment

At diagnosis, the primary care provider's office made an appointment for MG with the on-site RD. They gave MG the "Patient Questionnaire for Type 2 Diabetes" (Fig. 1, pages ix–x) from the *Nutrition Practice Guidelines for Type 1 and 2 Diabetes Mellitus* (see Resources) and instructed her to complete it before her appointment. The RD obtained MG's medical record for review before her appointment.

Review of MG's medical record indicated that this is her second visit to this clinic, she is obese (~60 lb overweight), and she has not sought any medical care over the past five years. At 62 inches tall and weighing 175 lb, she has a BMI of 33. Her blood pressure was 124/78 mmHg. Her primary care provider

Laboratory values in the chart include:		Reference range
A1C	8.1%	≤6.5%
Fasting blood glucose	179 mg/dl	65–109 mg/dl
Fasting lipid profile		
Triglycerides	420 mg/dl	0–199 mg/dl
Cholesterol, total	205 mg/dl	100–199 mg/dl
HDL	30 mg/dl	35–150 mg/dl
LDL	195 mg/dl	62–130 mg/dl
Chol/HDL ratio	6.84	2.0–4.5
Microalbumin	negative	

had evaluated her and recommended that MG incorporate moderate physical activity into her daily regimen.

The initial visit with the RD was scheduled for 90 minutes. At that time, the RD reviewed with MG the "Patient Questionnaire for Type 2 Diabetes" that she had completed and brought with her. The RD learned that MG was diagnosed with diabetes the previous week and was taking no medication. MG had never had nutrition education, and she was at her highest weight, which had been increasing for ~10 years. She had "dieted" over the years, but it "never seemed to do any good." MG indicated she would like to weigh 130 lb. Her appetite was good, and she had no problem eating or digesting her food.

MG is a college graduate, teaches English as a second language to adults, and works long hours, frequently 10 hours a day. During the workweek, she eats "on the go" in delis and fast food and full-service restaurants and dines on frozen entrees at home. She almost always "orders in" for lunch and eats with her co-workers. She lives alone, loves Mexican foods, and enjoys cooking; however, because of her work schedule, she only cooks on weekends. She occasionally has an alcoholic beverage on the weekend if she goes out with friends. She drinks sweetened soft drinks with her meals during the week in restaurants and does not engage in regular physical activity.

MG is very concerned about her diabetes diagnosis because her grandmother lost her vision as a result of diabetes and other family members with the disease have had problems with their feet. She is afraid the RD will "take away" all the foods she loves to eat and is very concerned that she may have to inject insulin.

Goal Setting and Nutrition Care Plan

The RD asked MG what she expects to accomplish this visit and what her goals are for diabetes self-care. MG responded that she wants to lose 45 lb because her primary care provider told her that, if she loses weight, she can probably control her diabetes without medication. MG requested a 1000-calorie diet so she can get started. It is clear that MG is in the action stage. It is important that she experience success if she is to maintain her momentum.

The RD responded that MG has great long-term goals, but suggested they break them down into manageable pieces that are reasonable, attainable, and measurable in the short term. For example, a 45-lb weight loss is a long-term goal that is best broken into 5-lb segments, because any amount of weight loss will be helpful to MG. The RD explained that research shows that the people who are most successful at attaining and main-taining weight loss are those who combine physical activity along with caloric restriction. The RD asked MG whether there is time in her day for 30 minutes of physical activity and explained that it does not have to be done all at once but could be broken into three 10-minute or two 15-minute segments. She also asked MG about initial dietary changes she would like to make.

MG decided that she would walk 30 minutes a day, three times a week, to start. She could do this at lunchtime. She also thought that she should give up her sweetened soda. She de-cided to substitute diet soda or water for sweetened soda at lunch during the workweek. The RD agreed that these were good short-term goals that could be measured and reported at the next visit.

The RD explained that the long-term goals would need to be supported by education, so that MG could incorporate appropriate behaviors into her lifestyle without "giving up" the Mexican food she loves so much.

The RD selected *The First Step in Diabetes Meal Planning* (see Resources) as the initial tool for MG because, even though MG is a college graduate and working professional, she is also very busy. The RD decided to concentrate on what MG needs to know, rather than what would be nice for her to know. The RD also consulted *Mexican American Ethnic and Regional Food Practices* (see Resources) manual as an additional reference.

Intervention

Although the goals MG made for the next two weeks were walking for 30 minutes three times a week and substituting diet soda or water for regular soda at lunch on work days, MG had several questions about food. The RD used the remainder of their time together to explain that healthy eating is the first step in taking care of diabetes. She explained to MG that even small changes in her choices can make a big difference, it is important to eat a wide variety of foods every day, and individuals who eat out frequently may not be eating enough fresh fruits and vegetables. MG tends to eat in restaurants; she decided she could analyze her menu selections and see whether it is possible to order fresh fruit and vegetables. It may be necessary to try a different way to incorporate these into her daily diet, perhaps by bringing a piece of fruit or raw vegetables from home to supplement her lunch at work. MG might also consider decreasing her portion size at lunch by splitting a meal with a co-worker.

MG and the RD discussed the diabetes food pyramid and why starchy vegetables are a part of the base. They also discussed the caloric density of the fats, sweets, and alcohol at the tip of the pyramid. The RD pointed out where Mexican foods fit on the pyramid—for example, ½ cup of fresh salsa is a vegetable—and offered suggestions on how to use less fat in preparing traditional dishes. Small changes, such as substituting boiled beans for refried beans, grilling instead of frying meat, using corn or fat-free flour tortillas in place of the higher-fat variety, will help MG reduce her caloric intake.

The RD concluded the visit by scheduling a follow-up appointment in two weeks. She also told MG that she can call or email her if she has questions that need immediate answers.

> **Initial visit: Goal setting**
> 1. I will walk for 30 minutes per day, three days per week.
> 2. I will substitute diet soda or water for sweetened soda at lunchtime.

Documentation and Communication

Documentation for each visit includes the date of the visit, patient's diagnosis, the reason for the visit, history, risk factors, assessment, intervention plan, rationale for treatment, progress, time spent including start and stop time, and provider signature. The patient's short- and long-term goals are also a part of the documentation. The NPGs have sample forms that can be used (Figs. 1–3, pages ix–xviii), or the RD can develop them. In this instance, because the RD is employed by the referral source, all that is necessary for communication is to place the "Nutrition Progress Notes" in the patient's chart.

Evaluation and Reassessment

MG returned for a fasting blood glucose (FBG) two weeks later and a follow-up visit with the RD three weeks later. Her fasting blood glucose was 110 mg/dl two weeks after her diagnosis. She had lost 3 lb since her first visit to the RD. MG reported that she was able to walk for 30 minutes three days each week. She is still struggling with her goal to give up sweetened soda, because she does not like the taste of diet soda. She said she liked water better than diet soda, and most days, that was what she drank with her lunch. Evaluation showed that MG is making appropriate progress. She needs further education to learn more about all aspects of diabetes management and setting realistic goals.

The RD congratulated MG on the improvement in her FBG and on her 3-lb weight loss. MG was disappointed that she had "only" lost 3 lb. The RD took this opportunity to reinforce the fact that even a small weight loss can make a positive difference in diabetes management. Weight loss is difficult and although MG had "only" lost 1 lb a week to date, any weight loss is positive. If her rate of weight loss slows, she should not get discouraged and may attempt to improve her weight loss by strategies such as increasing physical activity.

The remainder of the 30-minute visit was spent reviewing *The First Step in Diabetes Meal Planning,* answering questions about Mexican food preparation, and discussing the importance of the role of physical activity in attaining and maintaining weight loss. The RD recommended the book *Latino Diabetic Cooking* as a good source of recipes (see Resources).

A follow-up appointment was made for three months. The progressive nature of diabetes will be discussed with the patient at that time. MG was instructed to call if she encountered problems before the scheduled appointment.

> **3-week follow-up visit: Goal status**
> 1. Achieved goal.
> 2. Achieved goal.

Documentation and Communication

The RD completed the "Nutrition Progress Notes" from *Nutrition Practice Guidelines for Type 1 and Type 2 Diabetes Mellitus* (see Resources) for MG's chart.

3

Managing Type 2 Diabetes with Oral Medications (Starlix [Nateglinide], Glucophage [Metformin])

SG is a 65-year-old Caucasian female referred to the RD for medical nutrition therapy for type 2 diabetes.

Assessment

SG has been a patient at the Diabetes and Endocrine Clinic with a five-year history of type 2 diabetes. She has never attended diabetes education classes, because she was always "too busy" and "could not afford" the extra expense. SG is recently retired from her job as a saleswoman in a local department store and is now covered by Medicare, parts A and B.

SG's nurse practitioner has just started her on Starlix (nateglinide), evaluated her for and recommended moderate physical activity, and encouraged her to make an appointment with the dietitian. Medicare covers this service, and because SG is recently retired, her time is flexible.

Review of SG's medical record indicates that diabetes is her chief complaint and she sees her primary care provider at least

Laboratory values in the chart include:		Reference range
A1C	8.5%	≤6.5%
Fasting blood glucose	120 mg/dl	65–109 mg/dl
Fasting lipid profile		
Triglycerides	150 mg/dl	0–199 mg/dl
Cholesterol, total	217 mg/dl	100–199 mg/dl
HDL	35 mg/dl	35–150 mg/dl
LDL	162 mg/dl	62–130 mg/dl
Chol/HDL ratio	6.2	2.0–4.5
Microalbumin	negative	

once a year. Her A1C has increased from 7% to 8.5% since her last clinic visit one year ago. She has been taking Glucophage (metformin), 1000 mg twice a day, for the past three years. At 65 inches tall and 160 lb, her BMI is 27. Her blood pressure is 129/82 mmHg.

The initial visit with the RD was scheduled for 90 minutes. SG did not fill out the "Patient Questionnaire for Type 2 Diabetes" she received from the person who made her appointment because she had misplaced it. The RD asked about her previous diabetes education and learned that she had never had formal diabetes diet instruction but had been told to watch her sweets and lose weight.

SG lives with her husband; her children are married and live out of town. She and her husband share cooking and shopping responsibilities, and now that they are both retired, they tend to go out to a restaurant for breakfast or lunch at least twice a week. They go out to dinner regularly either in a restaurant or at the homes of friends and frequently entertain friends in their home. Food plays a major role in their social life. When they eat at home, they generally eat their largest meal around 1:00 or 2:00 p.m. and have a light supper in the evening. SG said she didn't understand why her A1C was so high. She had been checking her blood glucose before breakfast three or four times a week for the past year, and it never was higher than 7.2 mmol/L 130 mg/dl. SG said she was not a "sweets" eater and that her primary snack food was fruit. She always kept fresh fruit in the house and usually had some for dessert. Her appetite is good and has not changed in the recent past. She takes a multivita-min supplement and 1000 mg calcium daily. She has no his-tory of hypoglycemia. SG does not "exercise"; however, she does housework and takes care of the flowers in her yard.

Goal Setting and Nutrition Care Plan

The RD asked SG what her diabetes care goals are and what she would like to get from this appointment. SG said that she wants to be healthy so that she can enjoy her retirement with her hus-band. However, she does not want a restricted diet.

The RD began the instruction by addressing SG's concern about her elevated A1C. She explained that this test shows what is going on with the blood glucose throughout the day. It re-flects both fasting plasma glucose and glucose changes due to meals and can be considered an average. SG only checked her blood glucose in the morning, when she was fasting. The RD explained that many people with type 2 diabetes have postmeal hyperglycemia because they have lost their first-phase insulin re-sponse. She drew curves showing how blood glucose responds to food and how the pancreas releases insulin in response to el-evated blood glucose levels. She showed how the Starlix recently prescribed by her nurse practitioner would help with this prob-lem by boosting the secretion of endogenous insulin in response to food eaten.

→ Insulin Released After a meal.

The RD then suggested that, if SG's goal is to "be healthy," she needs to consider how her food choices and physical activ-ity affect her health. In addition to diabetes, SG is overweight and has elevated LDL cholesterol. The RD selected *Healthy Food Choices* (see Resources) as a tool to help SG because it pro-motes healthy eating and provides a good introduction to diabetes meal planning. She thought it would be useful for SG, because she is in the initial stage of diabetes meal planning even though she has had type 2 diabetes for over five years.

Intervention

The RD used *Healthy Food Choices* to introduce SG to the dia-betes Exchange Lists. She explained that similar foods are grouped because, in specific serving sizes, they provide similar amounts of nutrients. She concentrated on the lists that contain carbohydrate and explained that carbohydrate is the nutrient that has the most impact on blood glucose. She pointed out the foods that contain carbohydrate: starches, cereals, grains, breads, pasta, beans, starchy vegetables, fruits, vegetables, milk, yogurt, and other foods in addition to sweets.

She also told SG that, if she lost even a small amount of weight, it would help lower her blood glucose and LDL levels. The RD pointed out the portion sizes of the foods on each exchange list. She explained to SG that it is possible to lose weight by decreasing portion size and increasing physical activity. She used food models to ask SG about her typical portion sizes and to demonstrate appropriate amounts of food to eat. She also demonstrated portions with measuring cups and spoons. The RD showed SG how to estimate portion sizes in a restaurant using her hands, as follows. A serving the size of a clenched fist equals about 8 fluid ounces and can be used to estimate the amount of hot or cold beverages. A cupped hand holds a half cup serving, and a 3-oz serving of meat fish or poultry is about the size of the palm (or a deck of cards). She suggested that SG maintain food records in order to become more aware of her eating patterns and that she check her blood glucose two hours after eating to see how her new medication was working.

The RD stressed the importance of physical activity for attaining and maintaining good health. She asked SG whether she and her husband enjoyed going for a walk together. The RD reminded SG that she had the long-term goal of being healthy. Would she consider setting a short-term goal to work on for the next month? SG enthusiastically said she would begin walking every day and would record everything she ate. The RD suggested that this goal was too ambitious, and they negotiated the goal of walking three or four days a week and keeping food records for one week.

The RD made a follow-up appointment for SG in a month. She told SG to make contact by phone or email if she had concerns or questions in the meantime.

> **Initial visit: Goal setting**
> 1. I will walk 30 minutes per day, three to four days per week.
> 2. I will measure my food and beverage intake for one week, record the amounts, and bring the records to my next clinic appointment.

Documentation and Communication

The RD completed the "Nutrition Progress Notes" from the *Nutrition Practice Guidelines for Type 1 and Type 2 Diabetes Mellitus* (see Resources), including beginning, ending, and total time of the appointment; SG's short- and long-term goals; and the date of her next visit; and placed the note in SG's chart.

Follow-Up Visit (1 month after initial visit, 30 minutes)

SG returned in one month with her food records. She had completed records for eight days. They showed that she was not consistent in her day-to-day eating patterns. Breakfast varied from orange juice, pancakes, eggs, and sausage to coffee and a sweet roll. The time she ate breakfast varied as well, from 8:00 a.m. at home to 10:00 or 11:00 a.m. if she ate in a restaurant. Sometimes the midday meal was the largest and included salad, meat, fish, or poultry, vegetable, and a starch. On other days, it was a turkey or ham sandwich. The evening meal followed the same pattern. SG reported that recording what she ate made her very aware of the quantity of food she had been eating. She measured her food at some meals at home and used the guidelines the RD provided to estimate portion size when eating away from home. Her postprandial blood glucose ranged from 130 to 170 mg/dl. 7·2 – 9·4

The RD commended SG on her efforts. SG appeared to have grasped the exchange concepts, so it seemed appropriate to introduce the healthy food choices guidelines. These would benefit both SG and her husband. SG and the RD agreed that the two guidelines they would focus on were "watch serving sizes" and "be physically active."

SG said serving size was a problem. She typically ate a larger serving than the *Healthy Food Choices* pamphlet suggested. It was hard to cut down. The RD recommended she make gradual changes. For example, if she was currently eating an 8-oz serving of meat, she should reduce it to 6 oz, rather than aim for 3 or 4 oz. The gradual change would allow her to become accustomed to a smaller portion without feeling deprived.

SG reported that she had not met her goal of walking three or four days a week. However, she had walked two days each week since her visit. The RD replied that she had made a very good start and that changing behavior is very difficult. She suggested that SG try to add one more day of walking each week between now and her next appointment.

> **1-month follow-up visit: Goal status**
> 1. Walking 30 minutes per day, twice per week.
> 2. Achieved goal.

Evaluation and Reassessment

The RD reported that SG was making excellent progress. She was taking her medication as prescribed and making a valiant effort to reduce portion sizes and increase physical activity. She had lost 3 lb in one month. Her next appointment for laboratory blood work was scheduled in six weeks. It was evident that SG was making satisfactory progress. Her next appointment was scheduled in six months.

> **New goals**
> 1. I will increase my walking to three days per week.
> 2. I will reduce my portion sizes of meat from 8 ounces to 6 ounces.

Documentation and Communication

The RD updated the patient's "Nutrition Progress Notes" and placed it in SG's chart.

Managing Type 2 Diabetes with an Oral Hypoglycemic Medication (Glucovance [metformin/glyburide])

HW is a 52-year-old Caucasian male referred to the registered dietitian (RD) for medical nutrition therapy for type 2 diabetes mellitus.

Assessment

HW was referred to the RD by his family practice physician after a diagnosis of type 2 diabetes mellitus approximately six months ago. The referral form noted that HW had been blind for almost 10 years following an industrial accident in the workplace. His visual impairment limited his reading and mobility. When the RD called to confirm his appointment, she learned that HW's wife would be accompanying him to the visit.

Review of HW's medical record showed the RD that HW had been instructed by an RN/CDE in the technique of self-monitoring of blood glucose (SMBG) using a monitoring system specifically designed for individuals with visual impair-

Laboratory values in the chart include:		Reference range
A1C	9.2%	≤6.5%
Fasting blood glucose	180 mg/dl	65–109 mg/dl
Fasting lipid profile		
Triglycerides	88 mg/dl	0–199 mg/dl
Cholesterol, total	189 mg/dl	100–199 mg/dl
HDL	38 mg/dl	35–150 mg/dl
LDL	100 mg/dl	62–130 mg/dl
Chol/HDL ratio	4.98	2.0–4.5

ment. The RN/CDE had also taught HW about foot care, emphasizing nonvisual foot assessment. HW and his wife were scheduled to see the CDE again within the next three weeks.

At diagnosis of diabetes, HW's physician had begun him on metformin but, due to continuing elevated SMBG results, had recently switched him to Glucovance, a combination of metformin and glyburide. The remainder of HW's medical history was unremarkable except for hypercholesterolemia, which was being treated with Lipitor (atorvastatin), and hypertension, which had developed two years earlier and appeared to be successfully controlled with the ACE inhibitor Accupril (quinapril). His most recent blood pressure reading was 126/78 mmHg, and urine microalbumin testing results were 32 mcg/mg creatinine.

At 69 inches tall and weighing 185 lb, HW has a BMI of 27.3. He had maintained a healthy weight before his accident but found that the inactivity resulting from his blindness had led to a gradual weight gain over the past 10 years.

At the initial visit, which was scheduled for 90 minutes, the RD completed a further assessment of HW's nutrition and lifestyle. His wife had filled out the "Patient Questionnaire for Type 2 Diabetes" (Fig. 4, page 22) from the *Nutrition Practice Guidelines for Type 1 and 2 Diabetes Mellitus* (see Resources) for her husband and brought it to the visit.

HW had adapted well to his blindness, spending most days at home on his own while his wife worked as a church secretary. Most of HW's meals were eaten at home, but he and his wife enjoyed eating out at a local Italian restaurant every Friday evening. HW was able to prepare simple meals for himself using adaptive cooking devices such as a talking microwave oven that he learned about after working with a blindness rehabilitation instructor. A typical day's food intake for HW was approximately 3330 calories, with 362 g carbohydrate. HW prefers to sleep late, taking his medications and eating two microwavable sausage, egg, and cheese biscuits with black coffee at 10 a.m. Lunch at noon usually consists of soup and a sandwich with fruit and chips. HW likes to take a nap after lunch and then have a snack of sugar-free ice cream or "diabetic" cookies with milk. If his wife has to stay late at work, HW will heat a TV dinner and eat it accompanied by two or three slices of white bread. Otherwise, HW's wife cooks dinner when she arrives home, which usually consists of a meat with gravy, two vegetables, rice or potatoes, bread, and a dessert such as sugar-free Jello. HW often enjoys a bag of microwave "lite" popcorn as a snack before bed. He takes no herbal, vitamin, or mineral supplements. He does not smoke cigarettes or drink alcohol. HW mentioned that he occasionally feels shaky and anxious when he wakes from his afternoon nap, particularly if he has eaten a lighter than usual lunch.

Goal Setting and Nutrition Care Plan

HW stated that his goal was to control his diabetes by oral medications alone and to lose weight so he could improve his mobility. He felt that he was generally eating "healthy" foods but was unsure of how to manage portion sizes. On review of SMBG records stored in his monitor, the RD noted that HW was checking his blood glucose on a fasting basis each day and, since beginning Glucovance, most results were within the target range of 80–120 mg/dl. The RD felt that HW's nutrition plan needed to address the issues of carbohydrate and calorie control, portion sizes, and sodium modification. Because hypoglycemia appeared to be an issue, the RD also stressed that HW needed to modify his SMBG routine and learn more about the symptoms and treatment of hypoglycemia. HW, his wife, and

FIGURE 4: Diabetes Patient Questionnaire

1. When were you first told you had diabetes? _6 months ago_

   Have you had previous instruction on diet? ☐ yes ☒ no

   If yes, who provided the instruction? _n/a_

   When was this done? _n/a_

   Do you have a meal plan? ☐ yes ☒ no

   If yes, how many calories? _n/a_

   How much of the time are you able to follow it?

       0%–25%   25%–50%   50%–75%   75%–100%

2. Have you been told to follow any other diet restrictions? ☒ yes ☐ no

   If yes, please check which restrictions.

   ☐ low calorie   ☐ low cholesterol   ☐ low/salt/sodium   ☐ low protein

   ☐ low fat   ☐ high fiber   ☐ other: _limit sugar_

3. Has your weight changed in the last year? ☒ yes ☐ no

   If yes, describe the change. _gained 5 pounds_

   What is your height? _5' 9"_

   What is your usual weight? _185 pounds_

   What would you like to weigh? _155 pounds_

   What has been your highest weight? _185 pounds_

   If you now weigh less than your highest weight, how did you lose the weight?
   _n/a_

4. Rate your appetite: ☒ good ☐ fair ☐ poor

   Do you have any eating or digestion problems?

   ☐ chewing   ☐ swallowing   ☐ stomachache   ☐ diarrhea

   ☐ constipation ☐ other: _____

5. What are your usual work hours? _not working outside home_

6. What is your usual eating schedule and what did you eat in the last 24 hours?

   Time _10 am_ Breakfast or first meal _2 egg, sausage, and cheese biscuits, and black coffee_

   Time _____ Snack _none_

   Time _noon_ Lunch or second meal _tomato soup, bologna and cheese sandwich, potato chips, apple_

   Time _3 pm_ Snack _sugar-free ice cream_

   Time _6 pm_ Dinner or third meal _meat loaf, green beans, corn, mashed potatoes, bread/butter, sugar-free jello_

   Time _9 pm_ Snack _bar of light microwave popcorn_

7. Who prepares the meals? ☒ self ☒ spouse ☐ roommate ☐ other

   Are there any special considerations in family meal planning? _____
   Blind due to an accident for 10 years

FIGURE 4: Diabetes Patient Questionnaire (*continued*)

8. How often each week do you eat in restaurants, cafeterias, or away from home?

    Breakfast __0__ x/week   Lunch __0__ x/week   Dinner __1__ x/week

    What type of restaurant? __Italian__

9. Do you drink alcohol?   ☐ beer   ☐ wine   ☐ liquor   *no*

    How often? _____   How much? _____

10. How many times a week do you eat these foods?

    regular soda pop   __0__ x/week

    sweet roll/pastries   __0__ x/week

    candy, candy bars   __0__ x/week

    desserts—pie, cake   __0__ x/week

    ice cream/other   __7__ x/week

    frozen desserts   __0__ x/week

    cookies   __0__ x/week

    other _____   _____ x/week

11. Do you take vitamins or any other nutrition supplement?   ☐ yes   ☒ no

    If yes, please list. _____

12. Do you exercise now?   ☐ yes   ☒ no

    If yes, what do you do? _____

    How frequently? _____ x/week

    If no, what exercise would you consider?   ☒ walking   ☐ exercise class

    ☒ other: __golf__

    Do you have any limitations on exercise?   ☒ yes   ☐ no

    If yes, please describe. __blindness__

13. If the doctor recommends a change in your current eating habits, would this be difficult?   ☐ yes   ☒ no

    If yes, why? _____

14. What eating concerns do you have? __Want to lose weight__

15. What would you like to know more about?

    ☒ weight loss   ☒ exercise

    ☐ eating out   ☒ label reading

    ☐ alcohol use   ☐ sweeteners

    ☐ other: _____

16. What do you hope to accomplish or gain from this appointment?

    I would like to:

    ☒ improve blood glucose   ☐ get more information

    ☒ improve eating habits   ☒ start exercising

    ☒ lose weight   ☐ lower cholesterol/triglycerides

    ☐ other: _____

Adapted with permission from *ADA MNT Evidence Based Guides for Practice*, Chicago, IL: The American Dietetic Association, 2001.

the RD set a goal of recording food intake using accurate kitchen measurements at least one day each week between now and his next clinic visit. They also agreed to modify HW's pattern of SMBG checks to provide his health care team with more information about his glucose control.

Intervention

The RD selected *Exchange Lists for Meal Planning* (see Resources) for instructing HW and his wife on diabetes meal planning because this tool helps teach proper portion sizes. The RD used the standard version of the booklet during her instruction but noted that it was also available in both Braille and audiotape versions from the National Federation of the Blind (see Resources). The RD estimated HW's caloric needs based on his sedentary lifestyle and subtracted 500 calories to arrive at a suggested intake of ~2000 calories per day to promote a gradual weight loss. She divided his carbohydrate intake into three meals with 60 g carbohydrate at each meal and added two snacks, each containing 30 g carbohydrate.

To assist HW in correctly estimating portion sizes, the RD suggested that he and his wife measure the amount of food that was held in their most commonly used ladles, cups, and bowls. She advised them to find utensils, dishes, and cups in the appropriate serving sizes, for example 4-oz juice glasses or cereal bowls that hold 1½ cups. She also mentioned the availability of "talking" scales, which would assist HW in determining accurate weights of meats and baked goods such as bagels and muffins.

Because HW uses many convenience foods, his sodium intake was well above 2400 mg/day, the recommended goal for individuals with hypertension. The RD taught HW's wife the various label terms denoting lower-sodium food products, such as "unsalted," "no salt added," "reduced sodium," and "sodium free," and suggested that she select lower-sodium versions of her husband's favorite foods.

The RD noted that Glucovance has the potential to cause hypoglycemia. She suggested that, in addition to checking fasting blood glucose daily, HW add an SMBG check during the day to provide his diabetes care team with more information. Thus, HW would check and record his blood glucose fasting and before lunch on day 1, fasting and before supper on day 2, and fasting and before bedtime on day 3, then repeat the pattern. The RD then reviewed the symptoms and treatment of hypoglycemia. She suggested that if HW experiences symptoms of hypoglycemia, such as shakiness, confusion, sweatiness, irritability, fatigue, sudden hunger or personality change, he should check his blood glucose, if possible, and follow the treatment approaches recommended by the American Diabetes Association, as follows:

- If blood glucose is under 70 mg/dl, eat or drink something with about 15 g carbohydrate. Wait 15–20 minutes and check glucose again.
- If blood glucose remains below 70 mg/dl, repeat the treatment and check again in 15–20 minutes.
- If blood glucose still remains below 70 mg/dl, the health care team should be called or HW should proceed to the emergency room.

Once blood glucose is over 70 mg/dl, the RD suggested that HW stop eating or drinking carbohydrate-containing foods, even though he may still feel the symptoms of hypoglycemia, because more carbohydrate can result in high blood glucose for the remainder of the day. However, if his next meal is more than an hour away, he should eat a small snack, such as a piece of fruit. The RD reviewed foods that contain about 15 g carbohydrate, including 4 oz fruit juice or regular soft drink, 6–8 oz low-fat milk, or 2 Tbsp raisins. She also provided sample glucose tablets to use if needed.

HW and his wife were enthusiastic about the potential for improving his health through lifestyle changes and had several questions. The RD invited them to contact her if additional questions should arise at home before their next visit.

> **Initial visit: Goal setting**
> 1. I will measure my food and beverage intake one day per week, record the amounts, and bring the records to my next clinic appointment.
> 2. I will check my blood glucose levels on the following schedule:
>   Day 1: fasting and prelunch
>   Day 2: fasting and presupper
>   Day 3: fasting and prebedtime

Documentation and Communication

The RD completed the "Nutrition Assessment Form" (Fig. 5) and the "Nutrition Progress Notes" (Fig. 6) from the *Nutrition Practice Guidelines for Type 1 and Type 2 Diabetes Mellitus* (see Resources). She placed her note in HW's medical record and sent copies to his physician and RN/CDE, noting that a return appointment had been set for four weeks.

Follow-Up Visit (four weeks after first visit, 30 minutes)

HW made good progress following his meal and SMBG checking plan since seeing the RD. He had met his goal of recording accurate food intake once a week, and he shared those records with the RD at his follow-up visit. HW now weighed 179 lb. His SMBG checks had been done on an alternating basis as requested. Since beginning his calorie and carbohydrate controlled meal plan, HW had experienced several episodes of hypoglycemia, which he treated appropriately. As a consequence, his physician reduced his dosage of Glucovance. HW's wife had begun reading food labels more carefully, and they both expressed surprise at the amount of sodium and carbohydrate he had been consuming before their first session with the RD.

> **4-week follow-up visit: Goal status**
> 1. Achieved goal.
> 2. Achieved goal.

HW felt that he would like to include more physical activity in his daily routine to promote continued weight loss. After a medical evaluation, his physician encouraged him to begin a program of physical activity. HW had enjoyed golf when sighted and had made plans to work with an Orientation and Mobility Instructor in a blindness rehabilitation program to attempt to golf again. The RD also suggested several alternate forms of physical activity, such as walking with his wife outdoors and using a treadmill or stationary bike indoors. HW agreed to try to include 20–30 minutes of physical activity into his daily routine at least five days per week, preferably after lunch when the risk of hypoglycemia would be minimized.

> **New goal**
> 1. I will include 20–30 minutes of physical activity in my day five days per week.

Documentation and Communication

The RD completed the follow-up encounter portion of the "Nutrition Progress Notes" (Fig. 6), placing her note in HW's chart and sending copies to his physician and RN/CDE. She noted that no return appointment had been set but that HW and his wife were free to call her to schedule additional appointments as needed.

Evaluation and Reassessment

HW's physician continued to see him on a routine basis and forwarded the RD a copy of the medical record notes and laboratory results from his checkup six months after seeing the RD. The notes showed that HW had lost an additional 19 lb and

FIGURE 5: Diabetes Nutrition Assessment Form

Name HW   Age 52

Diagnosis of diabetes 2/02   Present diabetes treatment Glucovance

Medical history blindness   Other medications

hypertension, hyperlipidemia

Date 7-20-02 Initial visit

Dietitian CJ

Chart # 20-10-30-4

Physician Jones

Lab Data

A1C 9.2%   BG 180 mg/dl

Cholesterol 189 mg/dl   HDL-C 38 mg/dl

Triglycerides 88 mg/dl   LDL-C 100 mg/dl

BP 126/78   Microalbumin 32 mg

Target Goals

Target BGs 80 mg/dl to 120 mg/dl

Target A1C < 8 %

Other

SMBG: Frequency fasting a.m.   Times of day fasting   Method fingerstick

Medical clearance for exercise: Y (N)   Exercise limitations visually impaired, will check with physician

Time	Bkfst	Snack	Lunch	Snack	Dinner	Snack	Total servings/day	CHO (g)	Protein (g)	Fat (g)	Calories
Starch	2	0	2	1	2	2	9	15	3	1	80
Fruit	1	0	1	1	1	0	4	15			60
Milk	1	0	1	0	0	0	2	12	8	1	90
Veg	0	0	1	0	2	0	3	5	2		25
Meat/Sub	2	0	2	0	3	0	7		7	5(3)	75(55)
Fat	1	0	2	1	2	0	6			5	45
Other	57g CHO	0	62g CHO	30g CHO	55g CHO	30g CHO					
							Total g	234	98	76	Total =
							Calories	×4 936	×4 392	×9 684	2012
							%Kcal	47%	19%	34%	

Ht _69"_ _BMI =_ (_27.3_ %) Wt history _gradual gain over past 10 years_

Wt _185 #_ (%) Reasonable wt _160 #_

Estimated calorie expenditure + Activity factor = Total calorie needs _2000 cal/day_

History

Occupation _disabled_   Hours worked _n/a_

Lives with _wife_   Meal preparation _self, wife_

Hypoglycemia _yes – midafternoon_   Eating out _1/week, Italian_

Schedule changes/weekends/school schedule _stable schedule_

Exercise: type/frequency _sedentary_

Appetite/GI problems/allergies/intolerances _no problems_

Vitamin and mineral supplements _none_

Psychosocial/economic _adapted well to blindness; good support system; no economic concerns_

Assessment

Diagnosed type 2 6 mo ago; SMBG 1/day; sedentary;
excess CHO, cal, sodium. Occasional hypoglycemia

Goals (nutrition/exercise/SMBG)

2000 cal = 60 g CHO at each meal, 30 g CHO at 2 snacks.
Limit sodium to < 2400 mg/day, check SMBG 2x/day at alternating times. Patient to check with MD for exercise clearance.

© 1996 International Diabetes Center, Minneapolis, USA. Used with permission.

FIGURE 6: Diabetes Nutrition Progress Notes

Client's Name: _HW_
DOB: _2-7-30_
Other Diagnosis: _hypertension, hyperlipidemia_
Phone Number: _555-555-1212_
Gender: _M_
Ethnic Background (Optional): _____
Medical Record #: _2010304_
Referring Physician: _Jones_

Encounters outcome	Intervention provided to meet goal (intervention = self-management training plus client verbalizes/demonstrates)				Outcomes of Medical Nutrition Therapy (MNT) — Goal reached (√ indicates goal reached, follow with number 1–5 as indicated* e.g. √ -3, √ -5)			
Encounters	1 (60–90 min)	2 (30–45 min)	3 (30–45 min)	4 (30–45 min)	Date: 7-20-02 — 1 Value	Date: 8-18-02 — 2 Value	Date: 1-30-03 — 3 Value	Date: — 4 Value
Clinical Outcomes					Value	Value	Value	Value
Preprandial blood glucose (md/dL)	O	R			180 mg/dl			
Bedtime blood glucose (mg/dL)	O/R	O/R						
A1C (%)	O	R			9.2%		6.9%	
SMBG, % in target range	O/R	O			~75%		100%	
LDL-C (mg/dL)	O	R			100			
HDL-C (mg/dL)	O	R			38			
Triglycerides (mg/dL)	O	R			88			
Microalbumin (mcg/24 hr)	O/R	O			32 mcg	/	/	
Blood pressure	O	R			126/78			
Height ___ Weight/BMI					185#/27.3	179#	160#/23.7	
Hypo/hyperglycemic episodes	O	R			20 x/mo	7 x/mo	0 x/mo	x/mo
MNT Goal: _2000_ kcal _240_ g CHO total _60_ g CHO/meal _34_ % Fat					1950 kcal; 230 g CHO total; 60 g CHO meals; 32 % fat	2000 kcal; 234 g CHO total; 60 g CHO meals; 34 % fat	___ kcal; ___ g CHO total; ___ g CHO meals; ___ % fat	___ kcal; ___ g CHO total; ___ g CHO meals; ___ % fat
Adhere to appropriate meal pattern, exercise, and medication treatment; plan to maintain blood glucose and lipids within normal limits								

Behavioral Outcomes	7-20-02	8-18-02	7-30-03					
• Eats meals/snacks at appropriate times	3	√5	√4	1 2 3 4 5	1 2 3 4 5	1 2 3 4 5	1 2 3 4 5	1 2 3 4 5
• Chooses food and amounts per meal plan	2	√5	4	1 2 3 4 5	1 2 3 4 5	1 2 3 4 5	1 2 3 4 5	1 2 3 4 5
• Verbalizes sick-day management skills	n/r	n/r	n/r	1 2 3 4 5	1 2 3 4 5	1 2 3 4 5	1 2 3 4 5	1 2 3 4 5
• Manages signs and symptoms of hypoglycemia	2	√4	√5	1 2 3 4 5	1 2 3 4 5	1 2 3 4 5	1 2 3 4 5	1 2 3 4 5
• Accurately reads food labels	3	√5	√5	1 2 3 4 5	1 2 3 4 5	1 2 3 4 5	1 2 3 4 5	1 2 3 4 5
• Uses modified or modifies recipes to total fat/saturated fat/sodium	2	4	4	1 2 3 4 5	1 2 3 4 5	1 2 3 4 5	1 2 3 4 5	1 2 3 4 5
• Uses healthy cooking techniques	2	4	4	1 2 3 4 5	1 2 3 4 5	1 2 3 4 5	1 2 3 4 5	1 2 3 4 5
• Selects appropriately from restaurant menu	2	4	4	1 2 3 4 5	1 2 3 4 5	1 2 3 4 5	1 2 3 4 5	1 2 3 4 5
• Participates in aerobic activity per exercise prescription	1	√5	√5	1 2 3 4 5 ___ x/wk ___ min	1 2 3 4 5 ___ x/wk ___ min	1 2 3 4 5 ___ x/wk ___ min	1 2 3 4 5 ___ x/wk ___ min	1 2 3 4 5 ___ x/wk ___ min
• Limits alcohol use to 1-2 drinks/day	n/a	n/a	n/a	1 2 3 4 5 ___ svg	1 2 3 4 5 ___ svg	1 2 3 4 5 ___ svg	1 2 3 4 5 ___ svg	1 2 3 4 5 ___ svg
• Verbalizes importance of smoking cessation	n/a	n/a	n/a	1 2 3 4 5	1 2 3 4 5	1 2 3 4 5	1 2 3 4 5	1 2 3 4 5
• Modifies medication/food for activity/lifestyle	2	√5	√5	1 2 3 4 5	1 2 3 4 5	1 2 3 4 5	1 2 3 4 5	1 2 3 4 5
• Verbalizes potential food/drug interaction Drug	n/a	n/a	n/a	1 2 3 4 5 ___ dose ___ dose	1 2 3 4 5 ___ dose ___ dose	1 2 3 4 5 ___ dose ___ dose	1 2 3 4 5 ___ dose ___ dose	1 2 3 4 5 ___ dose ___ dose
*Overall Compliance Potential**								
Comprehension	5	5	5	1 2 3 4 5	1 2 3 4 5	1 2 3 4 5	1 2 3 4 5	1 2 3 4 5
Receptivity	5	5	5	1 2 3 4 5	1 2 3 4 5	1 2 3 4 5	1 2 3 4 5	1 2 3 4 5
Adherence	4	5	5	1 2 3 4 5	1 2 3 4 5	1 2 3 4 5	1 2 3 4 5	1 2 3 4 5

Intervention: D Discussed, R Reinforced/Reviewed, Not reviewed, Outcome achieved, N/A Not applicable
* Key for Compliance Potential and Overall Adherence Potential: 1=Never demonstrated, 2=Rarely demonstrated, 3=Sometimes demonstrated, 4=Often demonstrated, 5=Consistently demonstrated.

INITIAL ENCOUNTER Date: _7-20-02_

Beginning Time: _10 am_ Ending Time: _11:30 am_ Total Minutes: _90_

Comments: _diagnosed type 2 6 mo ago. Visually impaired._
Sedentary lifestyle, Glucovance, Lipitor, Accupril.
SMBG: 1/day. Diet high in CHO, cal, sodium.
Experiencing some hypoglycemia.

Client Goals: _Control diabetes by oral meds; lose weight_

Material Provided: _Exchange Lists for Meal Planning_

Next Visit: _8-18-02_ RD Signature: _CG, RD_

FOLLOWUP ENCOUNTER Date: _8-18-02_

Beginning Time: _1:30 pm_ Ending Time: _2:00 pm_ Total Minutes: _30_

Comments: _179 #_
Doing well. 6 # weight loss in past month.
Keeping food records 1 wk – brought in for review today.
Checking SMBG 2/day. Treating hypoglycemia
appropriately

Client Goals: _More physical activity after clearance from MD_

Material Provided: _None_

Next Visit: _RTC prn_ RD Signature: _CG, RD_

FOLLOWUP ENCOUNTER _Chart review_ Date: _1-30-03_

Beginning Time: _____ Ending Time: _____ Total Minutes: _____

Comments: _____
Per Dr. Jones note: weights 160 # BMI 23.7
Physically active with golf and walking.
SMBG within target almost 100% of time.
A1C 6.9% Discontinued Glucovance.

Client Goals: _Continue without glucovance; stress physical activity and meal plan._

Material Provided: _None_

Next Visit: _RTC prn_ RD Signature: _CG, RD_

FOLLOWUP ENCOUNTER Date: _____

Beginning Time: _____ Ending Time: _____ Total Minutes: _____

Comments: _____

Client Goals: _____

Material Provided: _____

Next Visit: _____ RD Signature: _____

Adapted with permission from *ADA MNT Evidence Based Guides for Practice: Nutrition Practice Guidelines for Type 1 and Type 2 Diabetes Mellitus*, Chicago, IL: The American Dietetic Association, 2001.

weighed ~160 lb; his BMI was 23.7. He was physically active on most days and had begun to participate in a regular golf league organized by Rehabilitation Services. HW's SMBG results were almost entirely within the target range of 80–120 mg/dl preprandially, and his most recent A1C was 6.9%. His blood pressure and blood lipid levels remained controlled. The physician had discontinued HW's oral diabetes medication on a trial basis, providing he continues to maintain his healthy approach to eating and physical activity.

Managing a Postcardiac Type 2 Diabetes Patient with Insulin

DN is a 67-year-old Caucasian male. A retired hospital administrator, he has been referred to the registered dietitian (RD) for medical nutrition therapy for type 2 diabetes and cardiovascular disease. He is recovering from cardiac bypass surgery.

Assessment

DN called the RD for an appointment, stating that his physician had referred him and he had the referral slip. DN said his physician wanted him to start insulin after he saw the RD. On inquiry, the RD learned that DN had a fax machine at home, so she faxed him the "Patient Questionnaire for Type 2 Diabetes" from the *Nutrition Practice Guidelines for Type 1 and Type 2 Diabetes Mellitus* (see Resources) and asked him to complete it before his appointment. The RD also asked DN to keep food records until his visit with her at the end of the week. She

Laboratory values in the chart include:		Reference range
A1C (result >1 year old)	7.5%	≤6.5%
Fasting blood glucose	146 mg/dl	65–109 mg/dl
Fasting lipid profile		
Triglycerides	132 mg/dl	0–199 mg/dl
Cholesterol, total	170 mg/dl	100–199 mg/dl
HDL	39 mg/dl	35–150 mg/dl
LDL	117 mg/dl	62–130 mg/dl
Chol/HDL ratio	4.36	2.0–4.5
Liver panel		
Albumin	3.5 g/dl	3.2–5.0 g/dl
Bilirubin, total	0.6 mg/dl	0.0–1.2 mg/dl
Bilirubin, direct	0.1 mg/dl	0.0–0.3 mg/dl
Alkaline phos.	71 IU/L	40–120 IU/L
ALT (SGPT)	13 IU/L	3–45 IU/L
AST (SGOT)	20 IU/L	3–45 IU/L
Microalbumin	negative	

learned that DN's wife did all the food shopping and cooking, so she suggested that his wife accompany him for his appointment. She also contacted the referring physician's office for DN's medical records.

Review of DN's medical records indicates that he had had coronary artery bypass surgery two weeks earlier after a previous angioplasty reoccluded. DN has a ten-year history of type 2 diabetes and had been taking Glucotrol (glypizide), Glucophage (metformin), Lipitor (atorvastatin), and Capoten (captopril). Physician orders indicated that DN was to discontinue the oral diabetes medications (Glucotrol and Glucophage) and begin Lantus (insulin glargine; 12 units at bedtime) and Humalog (insulin lispro; 5 units before breakfast, 6 units before lunch, and 6 units before dinner). DN was to see the dietitian to learn carbohydrate counting and how to adjust insulin. At 71 inches tall and 165 lb, DN has a BMI of 23. His blood pressure on his most recent office visit was 129/78 mmHg.

The laboratory report showed that the DN's FPG and LDL were elevated. The A1C was done over a year ago, too old to be relevant. The records showed his hypertension was under control.

The initial visit with the RD was scheduled for 60 minutes. On reviewing the patient questionnaire and food records, the RD learned that DN had attended diabetes education classes ten years ago when he was first diagnosed and had consulted with an RD at that time. He had learned about the Exchange Lists and was given a 2000-calorie diet; however, he didn't follow a meal plan but ate the "balanced" meals his wife prepared and occasionally ate in restaurants. His wife stated that she did not use sugar either in cooking or at the table. She was very careful to purchase only "sugar-free" products but had a much more difficult time with limiting cholesterol because both enjoyed eating red meat. He also enjoyed eggs for breakfast. However, since his recent surgery, they had been "good": all she was cooking was chicken and salmon, and DN was eating cereal in the morning. DN had lost 10 lb since his surgery; his weight had been stable for five years before surgery. The surgery had frightened DN and his wife, and they both wanted to make changes to improve DN's health.

Goal Setting and Nutrition Care Plan

On inquiry, DN said his goal was to "eat right" so he could keep his diabetes and heart disease under control and get off insulin and back on pills. The first thing the RD explained was the progressive nature of type 2 diabetes and the importance of improving glucose control using whatever means necessary. She said they would establish a measurable short-term goal before the end of today's appointment.

Although the nutrition care plan needs to address cholesterol, saturated fat, sodium, and carbohydrate counting, the RD suggested that they spend some time talking about the insulin the physician had ordered and how it interacts with food.

Intervention

The RD started by explaining insulin action. She noted that Lantus lasts a long time, which is why DN will take it only once a day, whereas Humalog acts quickly and is injected before each meal. She explained that carbohydrate is the nutrient that has the most impact on blood glucose and that carbohydrate counting is a good way to learn more about balancing insulin and food for glycemic control. She said that DN would be able to establish a ratio between the amount of carbohydrate he eats and the amount of insulin he injects before each meal, called an insulin-carbohydrate ratio. The RD went back to the food records DN had brought to this appointment. She pointed out the carbohydrate-containing foods and observed that DN had eaten a consistent amount of carbohydrate at breakfast each day, 70 g. The amount of carbohydrate eaten at lunch and dinner had been much more variable and ranged from 70 to 110 g. She gave DN and his wife a copy of the *Exchange Lists for Meal Planning* (see Resources) and reviewed with them the lists that contain foods with carbohydrate. She explained that the portions of food listed contain 15 g carbohydrate. The RD showed them how the Nutrition Facts panel on food labels can be used to obtain carbohydrate information. She alerted them that the information on the label is for one serving, and that it is important to check serving size. She inquired about measuring cups and spoons and learned they were available. DN's wife said she had a food scale, so they could weigh or measure all the food he ate. The RD asked DN to keep food records and to check and record his blood glucose two hours after each meal so that an accurate insulin-carbohydrate ratio could be established.

DN and the RD agreed that record keeping was an appropriate immediate goal, and they made an appointment to follow up in two weeks.

Initial visit: Goal setting
1. I will measure my food and beverage intake five days per week, record the amounts, and bring the records to my next clinic appointment.
2. I will check and record my blood glucose levels two hours after each meal.

Documentation and Communication

The RD completed the initial encounter portion of the "Nutrition Progress Notes" from the *Nutrition Practice Guidelines for Type 1 and Type 2 Diabetes Mellitus* (see Resources) for DN. She included a copy of these with a note thanking DN's physician for the referral and informing the physician that DN has a follow-up visit scheduled.

Follow-Up Visit (2 weeks after initial visit, 45 minutes)

DN returned in two weeks with food and SMBG records. The RD observed that DN had recorded most eating episodes and was quite faithful in recording the results of SMBG, so she commented that he had done a good job. It was obvious to the RD that DN was motivated to take care of his health at this point in his life. DN stated that taking insulin was not so bad after all because the needle on the pen injector was short and small.

2-week follow-up visit: Goal status
1. Achieved goal.
2. Achieved goal.

DN ate relatively consistently at breakfast: 4 oz orange juice, ⅔ cup raisin bran with 1 cup 1% milk, and black coffee on most days. Occasionally, he went out to breakfast and would have 8 oz juice, scrambled eggs, bacon, 2 slices toast, and coffee.

DN's basal insulin needs were covered by Lantus. By virtue of his consistent eating, it was apparent that his insulin-carbohydrate ratio at breakfast was 1:12. His eating pattern at lunch and dinner were more varied, with carbohydrate ranging from 75 to 110 g; however, a ratio of 1:15 looked reasonable to the RD.

The RD explained that with this information DN could adjust the amount of insulin he took before a meal, based on the amount of carbohydrate he planned to eat. For example, if he planned to eat 60 g carbohydrate at breakfast, he would inject 5 units Humalog, based on a 1:12 ratio at breakfast. If he wanted to eat 75 g carbohydrate, he would need 6 units. However, because his ratio is different at lunch (1:15), if he decided to eat 75 g carbohydrate at lunch, he would inject 5 units Humalog. The RD encouraged DN to continue record keeping and monitoring his blood glucose so that they could track and fine-tune his insulin-carbohydrate ratios. She recommended that he check his 2-hour postprandial blood glucose levels to verify that his insulin-carbohydrate ratio is accurate. Because insulin needs and insulin sensitivity may vary throughout the day, SMBG is the preferred way to monitor progress.

The RD then asked DN about cholesterol. She explained that cholesterol was found only in animal products, but that saturated fat in the diet affects serum cholesterol. She gave DN a brochure listing the amount of cholesterol and saturated fat in foods and recommended that DN aim for no more than 200 mg cholesterol per day because of his heart disease and his need to lower his cholesterol level. The RD also recommended that he limit saturated fat to less than 7% of total calories. She said that one way to start this process is to use more vegetable oils than solid fats in cooking. Olive oil and canola oil are both good sources of monounsaturated fat but like all fats they need to be eaten in moderation. She gave specific examples of foods to eat less of, such as high-fat meats and the skin of poultry, and said to eat no more than two egg yolks per week. She suggested that DN trim all visible fat from meat and select lean cuts when having red meat. She also recommended that DN select low- or nonfat dairy products.

Because DN is taking medication to control hypertension, the RD also addressed his sodium intake. DN does not need to severely limit sodium; his daily goal is 2400 milligrams. His wife enjoys cooking, and he seldom eats processed foods. The RD discussed sources of sodium and ways to decrease the amount of sodium used in cooking.

The RD asked DN to revisit his initial goal of getting off insulin. DN agreed that controlling his diabetes is his goal. He also wants to keep his cholesterol and blood pressure under control. The RD agreed with these long-term goals and asked DN what he wished to accomplish before his next visit. DN said he would continue to keep food records and monitor his blood glucose twice per day. A follow-up appointment was scheduled for one month. The RD requested that DN bring his food records with him at that time.

Documentation and Communication

The RD documented this visit on the follow-up encounter portion of the "Nutrition Progress Notes," including the date of the next visit, and sent a copy to DN's referring physician.

Evaluation and Reassessment (6 weeks after initial visit, 4 weeks after first follow-up)

DN returned for his third visit and said he had seen his physician a week earlier. His FBG was 89 mg/dl, and everyone was pleased with his progress to date. His weight was stable, and he was exercising four times a week in the cardiac rehabilitation unit. He had questions about how to count carbohydrate when he was in a restaurant or at a friend's home. His records showed that he was making reasonable food choices and that he was monitoring his blood glucose twice a day on most days. His blood glucose was within the target range of 80–120 mg/dl about 85% of the time. The RD commented that she was also pleased with DN's progress.

They spent the remainder of the time discussing eating out. The RD showed DN restaurant menus she kept in her office and helped him determine the amount of carbohydrate in some menu items. She also pointed out the higher- and lower-cholesterol choices on the menu.

A follow-up visit was scheduled for six months. DN and his wife were instructed to call with problems or questions.

Documentation and Communication

The RD documented this follow-up visit on the patient's "Nutrition Progress Notes," including the date of the next visit, and sent a copy to DN's referring physician.

Managing Type 2 Diabetes in an Adolescent

DM is a 13-year-old African-American male referred to the RD for medical nutrition therapy for type 2 diabetes.

Assessment

One week before DM's scheduled appointment, the RD obtained his medical record from his pediatrician for review. She noted from the history and physical notes that DM is an overweight adolescent whose mother had taken him to his pediatrician two weeks previously with complaints of fatigue, polydipsia, and mild polyuria. DM had always been "big" but had seemed to gain weight excessively as he went through puberty in the past year. At 67 inches and 160 lb, his BMI is 25, which is approximately 95th percentile for age and sex. DM's blood pressure is slightly elevated at 126/82 mmHg. His pediatrician noted the presence of acanthosis nigricans (a brown-black velvety-appearing darkening of the skin) at the back of DM's neck and in the folds of his skin. Both DM's mother and

Laboratory values in the chart include:		Pediatric reference range
A1C	9.5%	≤6.5%
Random blood glucose	255 mg/dl	140–160 mg/dl
Fasting lipid profile		
Triglycerides	138 mg/dl	0–199 mg/dl
Cholesterol, total	190 mg/dl	100–199 mg/dl
HDL	47 mg/dl	35–150 mg/dl
LDL	128 mg/dl	62–130 mg/dl
Islet cell autoantibodies	negative, indicating nonautoimmune diabetes	
Urinary ketones	negative	

grandmother have type 2 diabetes. The pediatrician felt that DM was at high risk for type 2 diabetes and obtained a number of laboratory tests:

Because DM presented with both a random blood glucose >200 mg/dl and signs and symptoms of diabetes, his pediatrician diagnosed type 2 diabetes. The pediatrician also noted that DM led a relatively sedentary lifestyle, although he did participate on the middle school football team. His diet consisted largely of fast food meals and high-fat/high-carbohydrate between-meal snacks. DM took no vitamins or medications on a regular basis.

DM and his mother attended his first visit with the RD, which was scheduled for 90 minutes. Both appeared interested in learning more about type 2 diabetes treatment and expressed a desire to avoid the renal complications and amputations experienced by other family members who had "bad" diabetes. The RD began by finding out more about DM's lifestyle, both at home and at school. She learned that DM lives with his mother and younger sister in a downtown apartment building. He is a very good student in 7th grade with a special interest in computers. His school does not offer daily physical education classes; however, DM participates on the middle school football team, which requires practice three days per week during the fall season. On most days at home after school, DM watches his sister, does his homework, and plays computer games until his mother comes home from her job as an aide in a local nursing home.

DM's diet recall revealed an intake of approximately 4900 calories per day, with 795 g carbohydrate; many of his calories came from foods high in saturated fat. On a typical school day, DM usually sleeps too late to allow time for breakfast. On those days, he drinks a regular soft drink and eats a package of peanut butter crackers while waiting for the bus to take him to school. If he has time for breakfast, it usually consists of two large bowls of sweetened cereal with whole milk, two or three chocolate doughnuts, and a large glass of orange drink. At school, DM often feels hungry and has two packages of snack cakes, plus a regular soft drink from the vending machine in the middle of the morning. A typical lunch consists of 3 pieces of pizza, an order of French fries, and a large carton of orange drink. If DM has football practice after school, he usually has 2 candy bars and a regular soft drink before practice begins; if he doesn't have practice, he goes home after school and has a snack of two bologna sandwiches, a "grab bag" of potato chips, and a regular soft drink. DM's mother arrives home from work at 6:30 p.m. She is often too tired to cook and stops at a fast food restaurant to bring supper home. DM generally has a double cheeseburger "value meal" with super-sized French fries and another regular soft drink. Before bed, DM likes to have a snack of cookies and a glass of orange drink.

Goal Setting and Nutrition Care Plan

The RD began by explaining basic information about type 2 diabetes in youth, emphasizing that the condition often begins during puberty when insulin resistance in combination with physical inactivity and excess calories leads to the diagnosis. She explained that treatment of type 2 diabetes in young people mainly involves lifestyle changes, which were most successful if the entire family participated in making those changes as well. DM's mother was willing to do things differently at home because she was concerned that her young daughter, who was already overweight, might develop diabetes too.

The RD reviewed treatment goals for youth with type 2 diabetes, including the need to normalize blood glucose and A1C, prevent complications, enhance lean muscle mass and decrease body fat, acquire and maintain healthy eating habits, and increase physical activity.

Because DM's mother was already comfortable with SMBG in her role as a nurse's aide, they both easily learned the procedure in their pediatrician's office. They set a goal of checking DM's blood glucose at least 3 times daily—fasting, after school, and before bedtime. DM was unwilling to do SMBG checks at school, because he didn't want to draw attention to himself and his condition. The RD offered reasonable target goals for whole blood glucose: 80–120 mg/dl preprandially and 140–160 mg/dl 2 hours postprandially. The RD suggested doing an occasional SMBG check before, then 2 hours after, a meal so that DM could see the relationship between his carbohydrate intake and blood glucose response.

The RD also explained that DM's lifestyle changes could improve both his elevated blood lipids and his high blood pressure. She estimated that removing 500–700 calories from DM's daily food intake would result in a gradual weight loss of 1–2 lb per week. The RD suggested that if DM would make the simple change of substituting water or diet soft drinks for his orange drink and regular soft drinks, he would avoid eating almost 1000 calories daily. She also pointed out the lack of fruit and vegetables in his meal plan and suggested that he "strive for five," beginning by adding a piece of fruit in the morning as well as to his after school snack. DM agreed to making these changes between now and his next clinic visit.

In terms of physical activity, the RD encouraged DM to participate in the upcoming football season, because 20–30 minutes of physical activity on most days would improve his blood glucose. She also mentioned that improving blood glucose would decrease DM's fatigue, leading to better athletic performance. The RD noted that it was important for DM to become more active at home and encouraged him to spend less time in front of the computer and television after school. She challenged him and his mother to think of ways to include more physical activity in his day, such as walking to school rather than riding the bus, helping with housework, or riding bicycles as a family activity on the weekend.

Intervention

The RD selected *The First Step in Diabetes Meal Planning* (see Resources) for instructing DM and his mother about food choices. She suggested that DM eat three meals each day with a snack after school and a snack before bed, emphasizing the carbohydrate content of each food group and advising DM to keep his carbohydrate intake consistent from day to day. They reviewed food label reading and proper portion sizes, as well as suggestions for healthier fast food choices. The RD again encouraged DM to increase his physical activity. He expressed a willingness to change, noting that he was tired of being "teased" by his peers because of his size. The RD invited DM and his mother to call her with any questions they might have. They scheduled a follow-up appointment for three weeks later. The RD asked DM to keep food records for three days before his next appointment and to bring them to their next visit.

Initial visit: Goal setting
1. I will check and record my blood glucose levels three times daily: fasting, after school, and at bedtime and bring them to my next clinic appointment.
2. I will substitute water or diet soda for orange drinks and sweetened soft drinks.
3. I will walk to and from school three days per week rather than ride the bus.

Documentation and Communication

The RD completed the "Nutrition Assessment Form" and the initial encounter section of the "Nutrition Progress Notes" from the *Nutrition Practice Guidelines for Type 1 and Type 2 Diabetes Mellitus* (see Resources). She placed her notes in DM's medical record and forwarded a copy to his pediatrician, informing him that a follow-up appointment had been set.

Follow-Up Visit (3 weeks after first visit, 45 minutes)

Although the RD left a reminder message on the family's answering machine, DM did not bring food or SMBG records to his clinic visit. He stated that his SMBGs were running 180–200 mg/dl fasting. He had also checked his blood glucose 2 hours after eating three slices of pizza and a regular soft drink and found it was 220 mg/dl. The RD commended DM on his weight loss of 3 lb in the past 3 weeks. She also noted that he had successfully substituted calorie-free beverages for high-calorie drinks. He was having difficulty with food choices at school. In addition to football practice, DM's mother had promoted a lifestyle change that resulted in increased physical activity: DM and his sister were now walking to his grandmother's house after school and helping her with yard work rather than staying indoors in their apartment.

3-week follow-up visit: Goal status
1. Unable to evaluate; patient did not bring records to clinic.
2. Achieved goal.
3. Achieved goal.

To teach DM more about portion and carbohydrate control, the RD presented him with *Exchange Lists for Meal Planning* (see Resources). She had personalized the materials to meet his energy requirements of approximately 2500 calories per day and carbohydrate targets of 80 g at each of three meals and 45 g at each of two snacks. DM set a goal of keeping his carbohydrate intake within the target range at least 5 days per week. He also agreed to send the RD a copy of the school cafeteria menu for the next month so she could make suggestions for healthy food choices and portion sizes. They scheduled a follow-up appointment for one month.

> **New goal**
> 1. I will limit my carbohydrate intake to 80 g of carbohydrate at each of my three meals and 45 g of carbohydrate at each of my two snacks at least five days per week.

Documentation and Communication

The RD documented the follow-up visit on the "Nutrition Progress Notes." She placed her note in DM's medical record and forwarded a copy to his pediatrician, informing him that a follow-up appointment had been set.

Evaluation and Reassessment

The RD saw DM and his mother on a regular basis over the next six months. His SMBG results were generally within the target range, except at times when he noted eating extra large portions of carbohydrate-containing foods. His blood lipids and blood pressure improved as he slowed his rate of weight gain. At the clinic visit six months after his diagnosis of type 2 diabetes, the pediatrician noted that DM, at 68 inches tall and weighing 162 lb, had a BMI of 24.7 (90–95 percentile). His random fasting blood glucose at that visit was 146 mg/dl, and his A1C had dropped to 7.2%. He was continuing to enjoy the health and social benefits of increased physical activity.

Managing a Type 1 Diabetes Patient with Celiac Disease Using an Insulin Pump

CR is a 35-year-old Caucasian female referred to the RD for medical nutrition therapy for type 1 diabetes.

Assessment

The RD had previously worked with CR when she was first diagnosed with type 1 diabetes at age 17. She continued to see CR when she was evaluated by the clinic endocrinologist and was placed on an insulin pump at age 26. Before CR's scheduled appointment, the RD obtained her medical record for review. She noted that CR had been diagnosed with celiac disease two weeks earlier after presenting to the clinic gastroenterologist for a gastroparesis work-up. CR had frequent bouts of diarrhea, which were felt to be due to gastroparesis or perhaps irritable bowel syndrome. At the time of her diagnosis with celiac disease, CR was 66 inches tall and weighed 117 lb and had a BMI of 18.9. The diagnosis of celiac disease was suspected after she tested positive for antigliadin and antiendomysial antibodies; an

Laboratory values in the chart include:		Reference range
A1C	7.2%	≤6.5%
Fasting blood glucose	93 mg/dl	65–109 mg/dl
Fasting lipid profile		
Triglycerides	66 mg/dl	0–199 mg/dl
Cholesterol, total	176 mg/dl	100–199 mg/dl
HDL	38 mg/dl	35–150 mg/dl
LDL	93 mg/dl	62–130 mg/dl
Chol/HDL ratio	4.64	2.0–4.5
Serum albumin	3.2 g/dl	3.5–5.0 g/dl
Prealbumin	17 mg/dl	19–43 mg/dl
Hemoglobin	10 mg/dl	1216 g/dl
Hematocrit	35%	37–47%
Microalbumin	negative	

intestinal biopsy confirmed the diagnosis. CR had depleted blood levels of iron, folate, and ferritin. She began treatment for iron deficiency anemia with a multivitamin with iron that also contained folate. Her calcium levels were also noted to be below normal, and for this she was receiving a calcium and vitamin D supplement each day.

CR was single, and her job as a pharmaceutical sales representative required her to keep a hectic schedule. After nine years of multiple daily injections, she wanted to try an insulin pump to allow more freedom in her lifestyle. At age 26, after an initial evaluation and pump training, CR made a good transition to insulin pump therapy, experiencing few problems until the past six months when she began having unexplained hypoglycemia followed by swings in blood glucose levels. Laboratory results in her medical record were dated one month before her visit with the RD.

At CR's initial visit, the RD learned more about CR's lifestyle and diabetes management skills. CR checks her blood glucose four times daily, fasting and before lunch, supper, and bedtime. She then adjusts her bolus dose of insulin based on her SMBG result and the amount of carbohydrate she anticipates eating.

CR's insulin-carbohydrate ratio is 1:15, so for every 15 g carbohydrate CR anticipates eating, she would include one unit of rapid-acting insulin in the bolus dose. Most of CR's SMBG results are within the target range of 80–120 mg/dl preprandially; she does not check her blood glucose postprandially unless she is having symptoms of hypoglycemia, which CR estimates occur once or twice weekly. CR treats hypoglycemia by eating animal crackers or drinking 4 oz orange juice; if she is driving, she eats two to three glucose tablets that she keeps in her glove compartment. As far as physical activity, CR works out with a friend at her local YMCA three times a week, usually walking on a treadmill for 40 minutes at each session.

CR has found it difficult to eat much, particularly during the weeks before her diagnosis with celiac disease; she often has diarrhea a few hours after eating a meal. Her diet recall revealed an intake of approximately 1050 calories with 150 grams of carbohydrate. She usually grabs a mini-bagel with low-fat cream cheese, a piece of fruit, and black coffee for breakfast; lunch is generally "on the road" and consists of a chef's salad with low-fat ranch dressing, two packages of crackers, and a diet drink. She often goes out to eat a late dinner with friends, choosing items such as pasta with tomato sauce or grilled chicken, salad, bread, and an occasional alcoholic beverage. CR told the RD that since her diagnosis of celiac disease, she has been afraid to eat much of anything and was quite discouraged by the number of foods that appeared "off limits" because of their gluten content.

Goal Setting and Nutrition Care Plan

The main concern for CR and the RD at this visit was incorporating the diet modifications required for celiac disease into CR's diabetes meal plan. The RD began by explaining the association between celiac disease and type 1 diabetes. CR's reaction to certain protein fractions in foods known as "prolamins" was causing damage to her intestinal mucosa, leading to the gastrointestinal symptoms she had been experiencing.

Although CR had been told she would be following a gluten-free diet, the offending prolamins are found not only in wheat gliadin, but also in grains such as barley, rye, and oats. The RD explained that CR should notice almost immediate improvement in her symptoms following the complete removal of gluten-containing foods from her diet. The RD and CR agreed that she would continue to adjust her bolus insulin dosage based on her SMBG results and anticipated carbohydrate intake. CR also agreed to keep detailed food records and to bring labels from foods she ate frequently to her next clinic visit.

Intervention

CR was already successfully using the carbohydrate counting approach to meal planning. It provided the flexibility CR would need to make gluten-free choices. Because CR's SMBG results were generally within target range, the RD suggested that she continue using an insulin-carbohydrate ratio of 1:15 and check her SMBG frequently during this period of adjustment. The RD also recommended that CR check a postprandial blood glucose occasionally. The RD modified the existing carbohydrate counting educational materials by marking through food sources of gluten such as wheat, rye, oats, barley, processed cheese, dairy foods, canned soups, luncheon meats, textured vegetable protein, noodle or pasta mixes, and ice cream. She also taught CR to evaluate food labels for gluten sources that might be found in thickening agents, modified food starch, mono-sodium glutamate, cereal fillers, malt extracts, distilled vinegar, emulsifiers, and stabilizers. The RD also suggested that CR check her vitamin and supplement labels to be sure they didn't contain gluten sources. The RD provided CR with several web sites for people with celiac disease (see Resources), as well as some suggested readings and cookbooks. CR felt overwhelmed and focused only on what she "couldn't have." Together, she and the RD planned a few days of sample menus based on "allowable" foods, which eased CR's anxiety. They scheduled a follow-up visit for two weeks later, and the RD invited CR to contact her with any questions that might arise in the interim.

Initial visit: Goal setting
1. I will measure my food and beverage intake five days per week, record the amounts, and bring the records to my next clinic appointment.
2. I will evaluate the labels from my food and vitamin products to identify sources of gluten.
3. I will check and record my blood glucose level four times daily (fasting, prelunch, presupper, and bedtime) and bring the results to my next clinic appointment.
4. I will check and record my 2-hour postprandial blood glucose level twice per week.

Documentation and Communication

The RD completed the initial encounter portion of the "Nutrition Practice Notes" from the *Nutrition Practice Guidelines for Type 1 and Type 2 Diabetes Mellitus* (see Resources). She placed her note in CR's medical record and sent a copy, with a thank you for the referral, to CR's physicians, noting that a follow-up appointment had been arranged.

Follow-Up Visit (2 weeks after first visit, 60 minutes)

The RD called CR to remind her of her upcoming clinic visit and was pleased to find that CR felt she was adjusting well to the changes in her meal plan. At her clinic visit, CR had gained 1 lb and reported a vast improvement in her gastrointestinal symptoms since beginning the gluten-free diet. Her food records indicated that she was eating three meals a day and an occasional snack consisting of foods such as plain meats, fish, fruits, vegetables, rice, and corn. CR stated that, if she avoided processed foods, she was generally better able to avoid gluten.

Her favorite snack was peanut butter spread on a rice cake with sliced apples. The RD noted several SMBG results that were out of target range after eating gluten-free bread and pasta products. CR explained that after reading the food labels of these products more closely, she realized they did not contain the standard amount of carbohydrate per serving she had been used to routinely counting. CR had only experienced one episode of hypoglycemia in the past two weeks and felt that was due to improved absorption of her food leading to better glycemic control.

> **2-week follow-up visit: Goal status**
> 1. Achieved goal.
> 2. Achieved goal.
> 3. Achieved goal.
> 4. Achieved goal.

CR and the RD spent time discussing strategies for restaurant dining on a gluten-free carbohydrate-controlled meal plan. As with eating away from home on any type of modified meal plan, the RD suggested that CR ask as many questions as necessary to determine whether a food was acceptable before ordering. Even eating a small amount of gluten from a grill that may have been contaminated with a few crumbs of wheat-containing food could cause a temporary return of symptoms. CR planned to call the headquarters of several of the fast food restaurants she ate in while on the road to determine which served foods that were gluten free. The RD praised CR's efforts and encouraged her to call with questions. She set her next clinic appointment for one month.

> **New goal**
> 1. I will contact three of my favorite fast food restaurants to learn about the gluten content of their foods.

Documentation and Communication

The RD completed the follow-up encounter portion of the "Nutrition Practice Notes." She placed her note in CR's medical record and sent a copy to CR's physicians, noting that a follow-up appointment had been arranged.

Evaluation and Reassessment

Because of a job promotion, CR traveled more frequently and was unable to keep her next two scheduled appointments. However, she did stop in to see the RD on the day of her six-month follow-up visit with the gastroenterologist. CR now weighed 130 lb, which at 65 inches tall, gave her a BMI of 21. She showed the RD her laboratory results, which indicated good nutritional status; she continued to take her multivitamin and mineral supplements. CR's fasting blood glucose was 99 mg/dl and her A1C was 7.1%. CR reported that she was an active participant in an on-line celiac support group, which provided a good source of recipes and tips for living with celiac disease.

Managing Gestational Diabetes Mellitus

MB is a 31-year-old Caucasian female referred to the RD for medical nutrition therapy for gestational diabetes mellitus (GDM).

Assessment

Within 48 hours of receiving the referral, the RD obtained MB's medical record for review and contacted her via telephone to ask her to begin keeping food records and made an appointment within one week for nutrition counseling.

Review of MB's medical record reveals that she is a healthy female who is in the 25th week of her second pregnancy. Her first baby was born at 40 weeks gestation after an uncomplicated pregnancy, weighing 8 lb, 15 oz. MB is 66 inches tall and weights 185 lb. Her prepregnancy weight was 175 lb (BMI 28).

Laboratory values in the medical record include the results of a 50-g glucose challenge test (GCT) performed at 24 weeks

8.6 mmol/L.

gestation. The one-hour blood glucose value was 155 mg/dl, indicating the need for an oral glucose tolerance test (OGTT). The results of a 100-g OGTT performed at 25 weeks gestation showed two abnormal values, confirming the diagnosis of GDM:

	Plasma glucose (mg/dl)		MB's values
Fasting	≥95	*5.2*	90
1 hour	≥180	*9.9*	230
2 hour	≥155	*8.6*	168
3 hour	≥140	*7.7*	136

Urine ketones at that visit were negative; an A1C test had not been performed. Hemoglobin, hematocrit, and blood pressure values were within normal limits for pregnancy.

The initial encounter with the RD was scheduled for 90 minutes. During that time, the RD completed a further assessment and found that MB lives with her husband, a police officer, and their 3-year-old son. MB has a family history of type 2 diabetes. She is concerned about the possibility of taking insulin injections and expressed her desire to "do whatever it takes" to control her blood glucose in order to have a healthy baby. MB does not smoke cigarettes or drink alcohol. She has no regular program of physical activity because she feels "too tired" after a long day at her job as a paralegal.

Diet Hx

MB's food records showed an intake of approximately 3500 calories with 425 g carbohydrate daily. MB had been experiencing intermittent nausea throughout the day and ate frequently because it made her feel better. She usually eats a breakfast of sweetened cereal, skim milk, fruit juice, and a sweet roll. At mid-morning, she has a snack consisting of a bag of potato chips from the vending machine. Lunch is often a fast food "value meal" with a regular soft drink. By midafternoon, MB is hungry again and shares a bag of microwave popcorn with a co-worker. Supper is usually late in the evening and often consists of a casserole-type dish served with a salad, bread, and dessert. MB has a bedtime snack every evening of a large bowl of mint chocolate chip ice cream. Since becoming pregnant, MB has stopped consuming caffeine. Her only medication is the prenatal vitamin with iron prescribed by her obstetrician.

Goal Setting and Nutrition Care Plan

The RD began by ensuring that MB understood the physiology of GDM and the importance of **managing elevated blood glucose levels to reduce the fetal risk of excessive size for gestational age.** The RD explained the need for frequent SMBG and the relationship between food intake and activity on blood glucose. She noted the suggested American Diabetes Association's recommended glucose target levels for whole blood glucose in GDM:

Whole blood glucose:		
Fasting	< 5·2 mmol/L	≤95 mg/dl
1 hour postprandial	< 7·7 (8)	≤140 mg/dl
2 hour postprandial	6·6	≤120 mg/dl

Handwritten margin notes: N I < 5·5 < 8

The RD also explained the role of urine ketone testing in GDM, stressing that morning urine ketone testing will be helpful in determining whether MB is consuming adequate calories and carbohydrate to ensure optimal growth and development of her baby.

MB set a goal of monitoring her blood glucose four times daily—fasting and 1 hour postprandially. She also agreed to check her urine for ketones each morning and record both SMBG and urine ketone test results in a logbook. The results could then be brought in, mailed, or faxed to the RD and MB's obstetrician for review and management changes as necessary each week.

The RD then explained the rationale for nutrition therapy for GDM and began to develop an individualized food plan for MB. The nutrition plan centered on carbohydrate, which is the primary nutrient affecting postprandial BG level. The goal for MB's plan was to provide a carbohydrate-controlled, consistent meal pattern that promoted adequate nutrition, appropriate weight gain, and normoglycemia while preventing ketones. Because the ideal amount of carbohydrate is different for each individual, the RD began by basing MB's meal plan on the fact that 40–45% of total calories should come from carbohydrate, with the understanding that this amount would be adjusted based on MB's needs and food preferences as well as outcome data such as weight gain, SMBG records, and ketone monitoring results.

Based on MB's prepregnancy weight and BMI, the RD recommended a 15- to 25-lb weight gain during the pregnancy, with the pattern of weight gain to be slightly less than 1 lb per week beginning with the second trimester. To achieve this goal, the RD estimated that MB would require 24 calories per kilogram of her prepregnancy weight for a total of ~1900 calories per day, with a total carbohydrate intake of 190–213 g daily. The carbohydrate intake would be spaced evenly throughout the day to better control blood glucose.

MB set a goal of consuming a carbohydrate-controlled meal plan each day, consisting of 30 g carbohydrate at breakfast, 15 g as a mid-morning snack, 60 g at lunch, 15 g as a midafternoon snack, 60 g at supper, and 15 g as a bedtime snack. MB agreed to record her food intake every day and include it with her records of SMBG and ketone monitoring results.

Intervention

The RD selected the carbohydrate counting approach for instructing MB about her food choices. She provided an individualized copy of *Basic Carbohydrate Counting* (see Resources) marked with MB's specific meal plan. The RD taught MB to read food labels to determine the total grams of carbohydrate in a serving of food; she also showed her additional resources for carbohydrate information (see Resources).

The RD noted that certain foods, such as dry processed cereal, fruit juice, and other highly refined products, might lead to a higher glycemic response, resulting in a higher elevation of post-prandial blood glucose values. She also explained to MB that in women with GDM, carbohydrate is generally less well tolerated at breakfast than other meals due to hormonal response and morning insulin resistance. MB's initial breakfast carbohydrate intake recommendation of 30 g may need to be altered based on the results of breakfast postprandial SMBG values.

MB had questions about the use of nonnutritive sweeteners during her pregnancy and the RD explained that research shows that aspartame, acesulfame-K, sucralose, and saccharin are safe to use during pregnancy, although moderation is advised. The RD encouraged MB to continue to limit her alcohol and caffeine intake and to speak with her obstetrician about beginning a regular program of physical activity such as walking, because regular aerobic exercise has been shown to improve maternal blood glucose levels. The RD reassured MB, who seemed somewhat overwhelmed, and invited her to call with any questions that may occur. They scheduled a follow-up appointment in one week to review records and answer questions.

Initial visit: Goal setting
1. I will check and record my blood glucose level four times daily (fasting and one hour after each meal) and bring the records to my next clinic visit.
2. I will check my urine for ketones each morning, record the results, and bring the records to my next clinic visit.
3. I will measure my food and beverage intake every day, record the amounts, and bring the records to my next clinic appointment.
4. I will limit my carbohydrate intake to 30 g of carbohydrate at breakfast, 15 g as a midmorning snack, 60 g at lunch, 15 g as a midafternoon snack, 60 g at supper and 15 g as a bedtime snack.

Documentation and Communication

The RD completed the initial encounter section of the "Nutrition Progress Notes" from the *Nutrition Practice Guide-*

FIGURE 7: Gestational Diabetes Nutrition Progress Notes

Client's Name: _____ Phone Number: _____

Medical Record #: _____ DOB: _____

Ethnic Background: _____ Referring Physician: _____

Outcomes of Medical Nutrition Therapy (MNT)

Expected outcome	Intervention provided to meet goal (intervention = self-management training plus client verbalizes/demonstrates)				Goal reached (Check indicates outcome achieved, follow with number 1–5 as indicated* e.g. √-3, √-5)			
	1	2	3	4**	Date 1 ___ min	Date 2 ___ min	Date 3 ___ min	Date 4 ___ min
Encounters	1	2	3	4**				
Clinical Outcomes								
• Fasting blood glucose (*mean*)					*Value*	*Value*	*Value*	*Value*
• 1 hour postpartum blood glucose (*mean*)								
• 2 hour postpartum blood glucose (*mean*)								
• A1C								
• Urine/blood ketones								
• Blood pressure								
• Weight								
*Knowledge and Behavioral Outcomes**								
• Understands and uses blood glucose meter					1 2 3 4 5	1 2 3 4 5	1 2 3 4 5	1 2 3 4 5
• Tests blood glucose					___ x/day	___ x/day	___ x/day	___ x/day
• Tests ketones					1 2 3 4 5	1 2 3 4 5	1 2 3 4 5	1 2 3 4 5
• Records food intake					1 2 3 4 5	1 2 3 4 5	1 2 3 4 5	1 2 3 4 5
• Verbalizes relationship of food, BG, and exercise					1 2 3 4 5	1 2 3 4 5	1 2 3 4 5	1 2 3 4 5

• Recognizes foods that contain carbohydrate		1 2 3 4 5	1 2 3 4 5	1 2 3 4 5	1 2 3 4 5
• Understands and demonstrates use of a meal planning system		1 2 3 4 5	1 2 3 4 5	1 2 3 4 5	1 2 3 4 5
• Following meal plan: Chooses appropriate foods and amounts for meals		1 2 3 4 5	1 2 3 4 5	1 2 3 4 5	1 2 3 4 5
• Chooses appropriate foods and amounts for meals		1 2 3 4 5	1 2 3 4 5	1 2 3 4 5	1 2 3 4 5
• Eats meals/snacks at designated times		1 2 3 4 5	1 2 3 4 5	1 2 3 4 5	1 2 3 4 5
• Verbalizes appropriate weight gain for pregnancy		1 2 3 4 5	1 2 3 4 5	1 2 3 4 5	1 2 3 4 5
• Takes prenatal vit/min supplement as prescribed		1 2 3 4 5	1 2 3 4 5	1 2 3 4 5	1 2 3 4 5
• Discontinues smoking/alcohol		1 2 3 4 5	1 2 3 4 5	1 2 3 4 5	1 2 3 4 5
• Accurately reads food labels		1 2 3 4 5	1 2 3 4 5	1 2 3 4 5	1 2 3 4 5
• Participates in regular activity per exercise plan		1 2 3 4 5	1 2 3 4 5	1 2 3 4 5	1 2 3 4 5
• If on insulin, verbalizes understanding of how to deal with hypoglycemia, sick days and importance of consistency		1 2 3 4 5	1 2 3 4 5	1 2 3 4 5	1 2 3 4 5
• Postpartum: Verbalizes benefit of breast feeding and strategies to prevent diabetes		1 2 3 4 5	1 2 3 4 5	1 2 3 4 5	1 2 3 4 5
*Overall Adherence Potential**					
• Comprehension		1 2 3 4 5	1 2 3 4 5	1 2 3 4 5	1 2 3 4 5
• Receptivity (readiness)		1 2 3 4 5	1 2 3 4 5	1 2 3 4 5	1 2 3 4 5
• Adherence		1 2 3 4 5	1 2 3 4 5	1 2 3 4 5	1 2 3 4 5

Intervention: D-Discussed, R-Reinforced/Reviewed, ≠ - Not reviewed, √ - Outcome achieved*, N/A - Not applicable.
* Key for Compliance Potential and Overall Adherence Potential: 1=Never demonstrated, 2=Rarely demonstrated, 3=Sometimes demonstrated, 4=Often demonstrated, 5=Consistently demonstrated. See documentation guidelines. Reproduce progress notes for *encounters 5-7.*

INITIAL ENCOUNTER　　　　　　　　　　　Date: _____

Beginning Time: _____ Ending Time: _____ Total Minutes: _____

Comments: _____

_____

_____

_____

_____

Client Goals: _____

Material Provided: _____

Next Visit: _____ RD Signature: _____

FOLLOWUP ENCOUNTER　　　　　　　　　　Date: _____

Beginning Time: _____ Ending Time: _____ Total Minutes: _____

Comments: _____

_____

_____

_____

_____

Client Goals: _____

Material Provided: _____

Next Visit: _____ RD Signature: _____

FOLLOWUP ENCOUNTER　　　　　　　　　　Date: _____

Beginning Time: _____ Ending Time: _____ Total Minutes: _____

Comments: _____

_____

_____

_____

_____

Client Goals: _____

Material Provided: _____

Next Visit: _____ RD Signature: _____

FOLLOWUP ENCOUNTER　　　　　　　　　　Date: _____

Beginning Time: _____ Ending Time: _____ Total Minutes: _____

Comments: _____

_____

_____

_____

_____

Client Goals: _____

Material Provided: _____

Next Visit: _____ RD Signature: _____

Adapted with permission from *Nutritional Practice Guidelines for Gestational Diabetes Mellitus.* Chicago, IL: The American Dietetic Association, 2001.

lines for Gestational Diabetes Mellitus (see Resources), including information such as actual time spent with patient, patient goals, and materials provided (Fig. 7). The RD placed her note in MB's medical record and forwarded a copy to MB's obstetrician, informing him that a follow-up appointment had been set.

Follow-Up Visit (1 week after first visit, 30 minutes)

MB returned to see the RD in a week, bringing with her records of food intake, SMBG, and ketone monitoring. She was in her 26th week of gestation and had gained 1 lb since her previous visit. MB had been able to achieve her goal of SMBG four times daily, with all results falling within the recommended treatment range. In addition, all morning urine ketone tests were negative.

MB had made major changes in her eating habits, particularly in the area of portion control of carbohydrate-containing foods. Her carbohydrate intake was very close to the targets she and the RD had developed. MB reported experiencing much less nausea than previously, although she was still feeling too fatigued after work to begin a walking program for physical activity. The RD answered MB's questions about the carbohydrate content of specific foods she enjoyed eating, and together they planned ideas for between-meal snacks that would be convenient for MB to take to work. The RD encouraged MB to continue her efforts and made a follow-up appointment for two weeks later.

1-week follow-up visit: Goal status
1. Achieved goal.
2. Achieved goal.
3. Achieved goal.
4. Achieved goal.

Documentation and Communication

The RD completed the follow-up encounter portion of the "Nutrition Progress Notes," noting that MB was following the treatment plan and achieving clinical goals. The RD placed her note in MB's medical record and forwarded a copy to MB's obstetrician, informing him that a follow-up appointment had been set.

Follow-Up Visit (2 weeks after second visit, 30 minutes)

MB returned to see the RD at 28 weeks gestation, with a weight gain of 3 lb during the past two weeks. Urine ketone tests were negative. The RD noted that two of the postprandial SMBG results during the past two weeks were above the target range; MB explained that she had eaten unusually large amounts of carbohydrate at those meals, which may have resulted in elevated SMBG results. The RD suggested that physical activity such as a walk after a larger-than-usual meal would assist in bringing the SMBG results within target range. The RD answered MB's questions about GDM and informed her that GDM indicates an increased risk for developing type 2 diabetes after delivery. The RD spent some time outlining diabetes prevention strategies to be put into place after the baby was born. MB agreed to continue her careful SMBG and record keeping, and a follow-up visit was set for three weeks later.

Documentation and Communication

The RD completed the follow-up encounter portion of the "Nutrition Progress Notes," noting that MB was generally following the treatment plan, yet having a bit of trouble achieving clinical goals due to large portions of carbohydrate-containing foods. The RD placed her note in MB's medical record and forwarded a copy to MB's obstetrician, informing him that a follow-up appointment had been set.

Follow-Up Visit (3 weeks after second visit, 30 minutes)

At 31 weeks gestation, MB returned to see the RD, having gained only 1 lb during the past three weeks. Her SMBG results were again elevated 1 hour postprandially (≥140 mg/dl) at least one time each week, and urine ketone test results indicated small amounts of ketones on most mornings. On reviewing MB's food records, the RD noted that MB had stopped eating her bedtime snack because she felt that it was causing the elevated SMBG results. The RD explained to MB that the ketosis she was experiencing was a result of inadequate calorie/carbohydrate intake and that ketonuria during GDM is positively associated with a lower IQ in offspring. She encouraged MB to resume her snack at bedtime and advised her to avoid excessive periods without eating. The RD mentioned that MB might need supplemental insulin to ensure the good health of her baby. Although MB was unhappy about that prospect, she agreed that she would do whatever was needed to have a healthy baby. A follow-up appointment was set for two weeks.

New goals
1. I will maintain appropriate blood glucose levels.
2. I will achieve a target of negative ketones in my morning urine six days per week.

Documentation and Communication

The RD completed the follow-up encounter portion of the "Nutrition Progress Notes," noting that MB had been unnecessarily limiting her calorie and carbohydrate intake and was experiencing ketosis and sporadic postprandial elevations of SMBG. She documented her recommendations and the potential need for insulin injections. The RD placed her note in MB's medical record and forwarded a copy to MB's obstetrician, informing him that a follow-up appointment had been set.

Follow-Up Phone Contact/Visit (one week after third visit, 15 minutes)

When MB faxed in her weekly records of food intake, SMBG, and ketone monitoring, the RD noted that three of the 1-hour postprandial SMBG values were greater than the suggested target value. She called MB and discussed the results and the importance on contacting MB's obstetrician. The RD then contacted MB's obstetrician, and together they made the decision that insulin therapy was necessary. MB returned to the physician's office, where she was instructed on the techniques of insulin injection therapy, the treatment of hypoglycemia, and the increased importance of a consistent meal plan.

Goal status for new goals
1. Did not achieve goal.
2. Did not achieve goal.

Evaluation and Reassessment

MB continued to visit the RD and her obstetrician on a weekly basis after beginning insulin therapy. She gained approximately 1 lb per week in a steady pattern. Her SMBG results remained within target range, ketone monitoring results were negative, and food records indicated that MB was meeting her carbohydrate intake targets. MB delivered a healthy baby boy weighing 8 lb, 2 oz at 39 weeks gestation and planned to breastfeed him for at least six months. Her SMBG results immediately returned to normal after delivery.

MB came back to the clinic at six weeks postpartum, and her lab work showed a normal fasting blood glucose level. She was counseled on her increased risk of developing GDM with subsequent pregnancies (recurrence rate of 30–65%) and type 2 diabetes later in life (incidence of 40–60%). Risk-reduction strategies, such as achieving and maintaining a healthy weight and daily physical activity, were encouraged. MB was advised to return to her family physician for blood glucose testing and screening for diabetes mellitus at least every three years and to seek medical attention should she develop symptoms of elevated blood glucose.

Resources

The following articles are American Diabetes Association recommendations and standards of care. Position statements published by the American Diabetes Association are viewable online at www.diabetes.org, accessible from the health care professionals' page. The complete collection of position statements is an annual supplement to the journal *Diabetes Care* titled Clinical Practice Recommendations and may be ordered online at http://store.diabetes.org or by phone at 1-800-232-6733.

American Diabetes Association: Standards of medical care for patients with diabetes mellitus (Position statement). *Diabetes Care* 25 (Suppl. 1):S33–49, 2002.

American Diabetes Association: Evidence-based nutrition principles and recommendations for the treatment and prevention of diabetes and related complications (Position statement). *Diabetes Care* 25 (Suppl. 1):S50–60, 2002.

American Diabetes Association: Gestational diabetes mellitus (Position statement). *Diabetes Care* 25 (Suppl. 1):S94–96, 2002.

American Diabetes Association: Type 2 diabetes in children and adolescents (Consensus statement). *Diabetes Care* 23:381–89, 2000.

The books and resources published by the American Diabetes Association listed below may be ordered online at http://store.diabetes.org or by phone at 1-800-232-6733. Resources published by the American Dietetic Association may be ordered online at www.eatright.org. Resources copublished by the American Diabetes Association and the American Dietetic Association can be ordered through either association.

American Dietetic Association: *Nutrition Practice Guidelines for Type 1 and Type 2 Diabetes Mellitus.* Chicago, IL: American Dietetic Association, 2001.

American Dietetic Association: *Nutrition Practice Guidelines for Gestational Diabetes Mellitus.* Chicago, IL: American Dietetic Association, 2001.

American Diabetes Association/American Dietetic Association: *The First Step in Diabetes Meal Planning.* Alexandria, VA: American Diabetes Association, and Chicago, IL: American Dietetic Association, 2003. (Available January 2003.)

American Diabetes Association/American Dietetic Association: *Exchange Lists for Meal Planning.* Alexandria, VA: American Diabetes Association, and Chicago, IL: American Dietetic Association, 2003. (Available January 2003.) Also available in Braille and on audiotape from the National Federation of the Blind; call 410-659-9314.

American Diabetes Association/American Dietetic Association: *Healthy Food Choices.* Alexandria, VA: American Diabetes Association, and Chicago, IL: American Dietetic Association, 2003. (Available January 2003.)

American Diabetes Association/American Dietetic Association. *Basic Carbohydrate Counting.* Alexandria, VA: American Diabetes Association, and Chicago, IL: American Dietetic Association, 2003. (Available January 2003.)

American Diabetes Association/American Dietetic Association. *Advanced Carbohydrate Counting.* Alexandria, VA: American

Diabetes Association, and Chicago, IL: American Dietetic Association, 2003. (Available January 2003.)

Ethnic and Regional Food Practices: A series developed by Diabetes Care and Education Dietetic Practice Group of the American Dietetic Association. Chicago, IL: The American Dietetic Association, and Alexandria, VA: American Diabetes Association. Various publication dates. Titles available from the American Dietetic Association: Alaska Native, Chinese American, Filipino American, Hmong American, Indian and Pakistan, Jewish, Mexican American, Navajo, and Northern Plains Indian.

Leontos C: *What to Eat When You Get Diabetes*. New York: Wiley, 2000.

Leontos C, Mitchell D, Weicker K: *The Diabetes Holiday Cookbook*. New York: Wiley, 2002.

Geil PB, Holzmeister LA: *101 Nutrition Tips for People with Diabetes*. Alexandria, VA: American Diabetes Association, 2001.

Franz MJ, Reader D, Monk A: *Implementing Group and Individual Medical Nutrition Therapy for Diabetes*. Alexandria, VA: American Diabetes Association, 2002.

Williams AS: Teaching non-visual diabetes self-care: choosing appropriate tools and techniques for visually impaired individuals. *Diabetes Spectrum* 10:28–134, 1997.

Inman-Felton A: Overview of gluten-sensitive enteropathy (celiac sprue). *J Am Diet Assoc* 99:352–62, 1999.

Gaines FE, Weaver R: *The New Soul Food Cookbook for People with Diabetes*. Alexandria, VA: American Diabetes Association, 1999.

Fusté OV: *Cocinando para Latinos con Diabetes (Diabetic Cooking for Latinos)*. Alexandria, VA: American Diabetes Association, 2002.

Web sites

www.niddk.nih.gov/health/digest/pubs/celiac/—NIH information on celiac disease.

www.csaceliacs.org—Celiac Sprue Association/United States of America, Inc.

www.celiac.com—Celiac Disease & Gluten-Free Diet Support Page.

www.nfb.org—National Federation of the Blind.

About the American Diabetes Association

The American Diabetes Association is the nation's leading voluntary health organization supporting diabetes research, information, and advocacy. Its mission is to prevent and cure diabetes and to improve the lives of all people affected by diabetes. The American Diabetes Association is the leading publisher of comprehensive diabetes information. Its huge library of practical and authoritative books for people with diabetes covers every aspect of self-care—cooking and nutrition, fitness, weight control, medications, complications, emotional issues, and general self-care.

To order American Diabetes Association books: Call 1-800-232-6733. Or log on to http://store.diabetes.org

To join the American Diabetes Association: Call 1-800-806-7801. www.diabetes.org/membership

For more information about diabetes or ADA programs and services: Call 1-800-342-2383. E-mail: Customerservice@diabetes.org or log on to www.diabetes.org

To locate an ADA/NCQA Recognized Provider of quality diabetes care in your area: www.ncqa.org/dprp/

To find an ADA Recognized Education Program in your area: Call 1-888-232-0822. www.diabetes.org/recognition/education.asp

To join the fight to increase funding for diabetes research, end discrimination, and improve insurance coverage: Call 1-800-342-2383. www.diabetes.org/advocacy

To find out how you can get involved with the programs in your community: Call 1-800-342-2383. See below for program Web addresses.

- *American Diabetes Month:* Educational activities aimed at those diagnosed with diabetes—month of November. www.diabetes.org/ADM
- *American Diabetes Alert:* Annual public awareness campaign to find the undiagnosed—held the fourth Tuesday in March. www.diabetes.org/alert
- *The Diabetes Assistance & Resources Program (DAR):* diabetes awareness program targeted to the Latino community. www.diabetes.org/DAR
- *African American Program:* diabetes awareness program targeted to the African American community. www.diabetes.org/africanamerican
- *Awakening the Spirit: Pathways to Diabetes Prevention & Control:* diabetes awareness program targeted to the Native American community. www.diabetes.org/awakening

To find out about an important research project regarding type 2 diabetes: www.diabetes.org/ada/research.asp

To obtain information on making a planned gift or charitable bequest: Call 1-888-700-7029. www.diabetes.org/ada/plan.asp

To make a donation or memorial contribution: Call 1-800-342-2383. www.diabetes.org/ada/cont.asp